GETTING READY FOR BABY

KW-053-720

Daphne Metland

W. Foulsham & Co. Ltd.
London ● New York ● Toronto ● Cape Town ● Sydney

W. Foulsham & Company Limited
Yeovil Road, Slough, Berkshire, SL1 4JH

ISBN 0–572–01416–3

Printed in Great Britain at St. Edmundsbury Press,
Bury St. Edmunds.

GETTING READY FOR BABY

CONTENTS

INTRODUCTION

Tradition has it that all new babies do is eat, sleep and use up vast amounts of nappies. New parents soon discover they do far more than that! There's crying for a start, and smiling, and being sociable, and getting nappy rash, or growing teeth. There's a lot to looking after a new baby. No one can teach you how to be a parent. You have to learn as you go along. Being well equipped helps, and so does spending time with other parents who can usually pass on tips and hints. Often, though, these tips come too late. Only after you have spent three weeks trying to get nappies to stay on, does someone suggest a new way to fold them, or button-under vests which will hold almost any nappy on.

The same principle applies to baby equipment. If you have never pushed a pram it's difficult to choose one. It's only after your baby is born you realise that the sling you bought can only be used when there is someone around to help you tie it at the back!

Much of the information in this book has been discovered by my Testing Panel for *Mother* magazine. Each month we try out a selection of baby equipment and report on the results in the magazine. Many of the tips and hints have come from the parents in my antenatal classes. I teach these for the National Childbirth Trust, so I regularly meet expectant parents and continue to see them after their babies are born, so I have constant feedback on how different types of equipment wear and perform.

Throughout this book I have referred to the baby as 'he'. The choice of he/she was decided purely on the toss of a coin, and I apologise to baby girls everywhere, including my own daughter, for the use of the male pronoun.

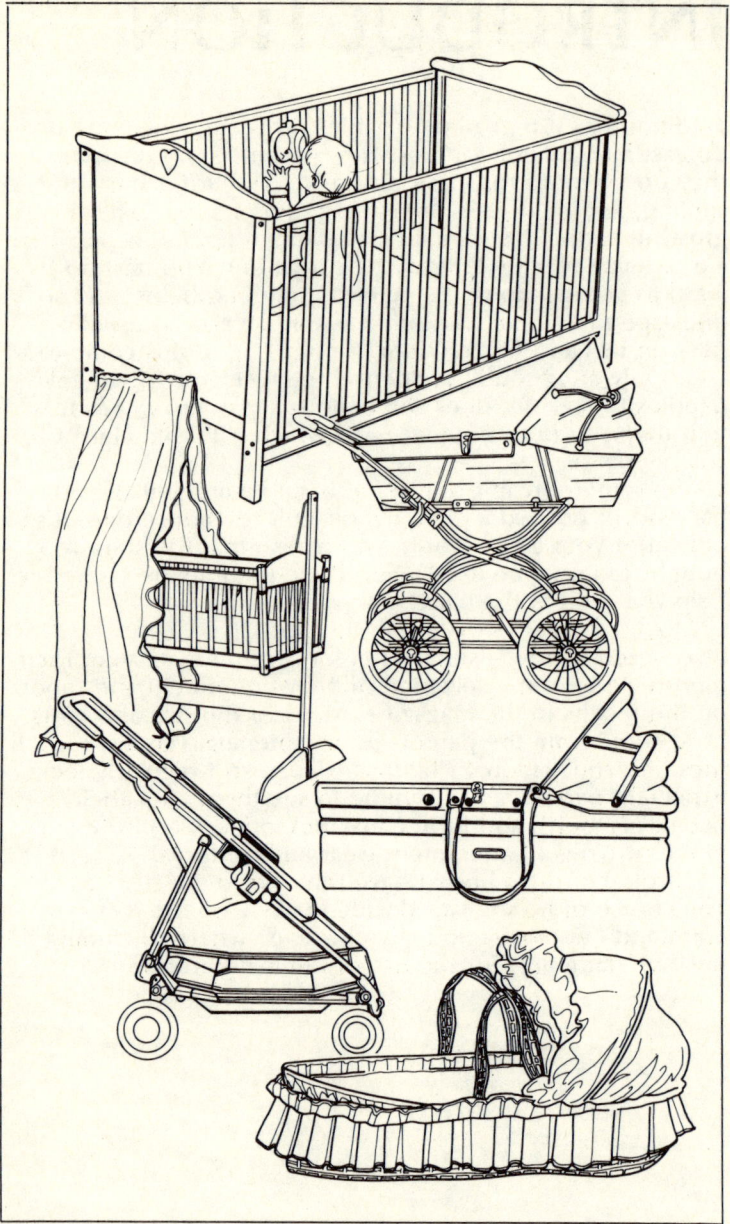

1 BEFORE THE ARRIVAL

Planning for a new baby does not necessarily mean rushing out and buying everything you see in the baby shops. If you do that you will spend a great deal of money, much of it on things you may never use. So it pays to do a little thinking ahead. Look round the babycare shops or check their catalogues, read this book, and decide on the essentials. Once you have those, the rest can be purchased as and when you need things, either direct from the shops or through mail order services.

You may also find that you are given presents for the baby, or asked what you would like, and most people are only too happy to buy something they know you will use and appreciate, rather than taking a guess at what to buy.

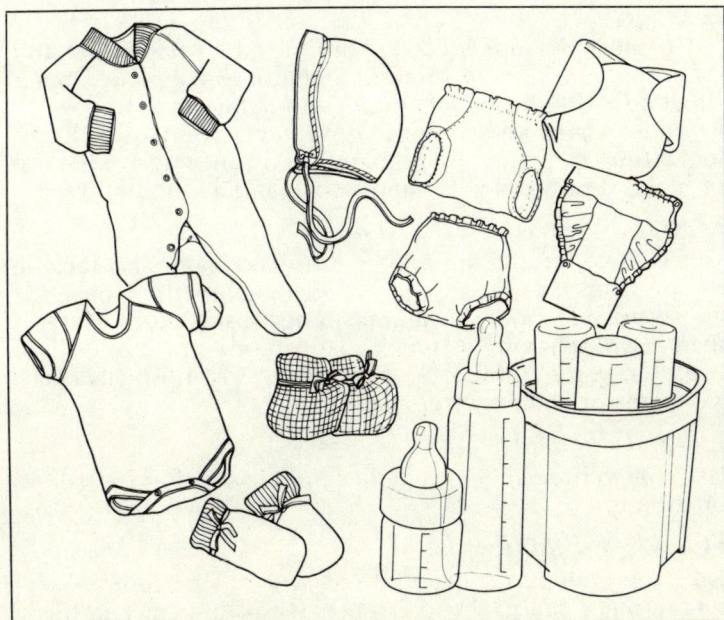

WHAT YOU NEED FOR THE HOSPITAL

It is a good idea to pack your hospital bags well in advance so they are ready and waiting when the time comes. After all, the baby may arrive earlier than you expect. Separate bags of the things you will need in the labour room, in the hospital, for the father, and for the baby are a good idea, so that everything is easily accessible and to hand at the right time.

HOSPITAL BAG FOR MOTHER IN LABOUR

In some hospitals your main case may be moved across to the postnatal ward well ahead of you, so pack a separate bag to keep with you in labour.

CLOTHING

An old nighty or a loose cotton shirt is comfortable to wear during labour. A man's shirt with tails is ideal as it covers most of your body but is loose enough not to restrict your movements. Choose an old one that is soft after many washings.

Hospitals do supply gowns, but they are often paper and they split as you move around. Linen ones have often been starched in the hospital laundry, and many seem to have lost their tapes. Remember that whatever you wear is likely to become soiled, so be prepared to throw it away after use or make sure it can withstand a soak and a long hot wash.

LARGE NATURAL SPONGE

This is ideal for dipping into cold or iced water and sucking during labour, especially for the shallow breathing needed for advanced labour. A natural sponge tastes much better than a synthetic one. Choose a largish one as it can be used for washing the baby afterwards. Most hospitals have ice cubes or chilled water available.

LIP SALVE

Use this to prevent your lips becoming sore during shallow breathing.

FOCUS OBJECT

Take something to concentrate on while using your relaxation technique. You can manage with a crack in the wall or the clock in the labour room, but something pleasing to the eye is preferable. Try a flower, an onyx egg or a small picture in a pretty frame.

HAIRBRUSH, SLIDES OR RIBBON

You may need these to tie back long hair as labour progresses.

CASSETTE TAPES

Take relaxing music to listen to while in labour. Practise relaxation at home to this music so you are used to relaxing to it. Check with your hospital if they have a portable cassette player. If not, you may need to borrow one to take with you.

MASSAGE OIL OR BABY LOTION

Massage helps a great deal in labour, especially for backache. Done for long periods it can cause friction burns, so use massage oil to prevent this. Use firm massage on the back, and gentle stroking massage around the lower abdomen.

FLANNEL

A flannel is useful to wash your face during labour. Choose a really soft fluffy one as the sense of touch becomes very important in labour.

TOOTHPASTE AND TOOTHBRUSH

In a long labour, cleaning your teeth can be refreshing. Also if a caesarian section seems a possibility, the labouring woman is not usually allowed to eat or drink. Cleaning your teeth can help you feel a little better.

HOT WATER BOTTLE WITH COVER

Warmth is useful to alleviate backache. Use a cover or wrap a cot sheet around the bottle to prevent it burning your skin.

MIRROR

Take a mirror to use to see the baby's head in second stage. Often being able to sit up with a mirror placed on the bed allows you to see your baby's hair at the peak of contractions. It's encouraging if the second stage takes a long time.

GENERAL BAG FOR HOSPITAL

Nightdress, dressing gown and slippers. Remember many hospitals are hot so choose a cool nightdress, and one in which you can breast feed the baby.

Feeding bras and a cream for sore nipples. Try a homoeopathic cream, such as Kamillosan or Chamomile as these do not need washing off before feeds.

Washing things including soap, flannel, toothbrush and toothpaste, one large and one small towel, hairbrush, shampoo and deodorant. Also take your make-up bag, perfume etc. and salt to add to the bath.

Books or magazines to read. Magazines are often best as you may not be able to concentrate for long periods.

Writing paper, envelopes, pen, stamps, address book, birth announcement cards. Also coins for the telephone.

Hair dryer or curling tongs. Many hospitals have dryers of their own. Often they insist that any electrical appliances are checked for safety before use.

Sanitary towels and pants (disposable pants are useful and save washing).

HOSPITAL BAG FOR BABY

Disposable nappies (some hospitals supply these), tissues, cotton wool, liquid soap for bathing, petroleum jelly.

Clothes to wear home. (Arrange for your partner to bring these in when he comes to collect you.) Most hospitals supply clothes while the baby is in the hospital.

HOSPITAL BAG FOR FATHER/LABOUR PARTNER

Flask tea/coffee/cold drinks. Snackfoods: biscuits/fruit/chocolate bars.

List of telephone numbers and change for the telephone. Camera with fast film.

Cotton short-sleeved T-shirt as labour rooms tend to be hot.

Note pad and pencil for labour log.

DAILY SUPPLIES

Often hospital food needs supplementing or varying. A wholefood diet and plenty of fluids are essential for new mothers to avoid constipation. Ask your visitors to bring in supplies along with presents for the baby.

Here are some things you might like to suggest: fresh fruits; bran biscuits; fruit juices; bottled water.

Extra small change for telephones, stamps, writing paper and clean nightdresses may also be needed.

You will also need your partner to bring in your own clothes to wear home.

THINGS TO DO AT THE LAST MINUTE

Before the baby arrives it's wise to stock up on some basic items and get certain jobs out of the way.

1. Fill the freezer. Make sure you have ample supplies of easy-to-cook meals. If you have time, stock up on home-made casseroles, pies, quiches and other dishes that are ready to reheat in the oven. If time is short buy some ready-prepared meals instead. Add some loaves of bread and frozen vegetables too. Try to organise things so that you won't starve if you don't have the time to go to the shops or the energy to peel potatoes.

2. Stock up on household basics: toilet rolls, kitchen rolls, canned foods, coffee, tea, etc. Try to keep a month's supply in the house to minimise the shopping you will need to do once the baby arrives.

3. Write a list of 'just in case' phone numbers to pin by the phone. Include your midwife, GP, hospital, partner's work number, the numbers of friends or neighbours who will drive you to hospital if your partner is unavailable.

4. Buy extra notepaper, envelopes and stamps for writing letters from your hospital bed. Buy some birth announcement cards if you wish.

5. Indulge yourself a little with a shopping spree for personal items like make-up, perfume, shampoo, conditioner, etc. Then you won't run out in the first couple of weeks when you often don't have the time to shop but want to look your best for all those visitors and photographs.

6. Sort out the baby clothes and leave some ready in the drawer for the day you bring baby home.

7. Decide what you plan to wear home from hospital. Choose something loose as you are unlikely to fit into your jeans! Make sure your partner knows what to bring in to hospital for you. Leave a list if necessary.
8. Think about using the Family Allowance that you will receive once the baby is born to make the first few weeks easier. It may be worth paying someone to help with the housework for a few weeks, or simply pay a teenager to do the ironing. Generally the Family Allowance will cover the cost of disposable nappies, or an occasional 'take-away' meal as a treat for the new parents.
9. Make up a bag of food for your labour partner. Freeze some sandwiches and try to remember to put them in your bag to take to the hospital.
10. Make an appointment to have you hair cut about two weeks before the baby is due.
11. Write a list of things to do if you are overdue. It becomes very boring sitting at home and answering the telephone. Try to have something specific to do each day. You may like to include some of the following:
Visit the chiropodist (it's usually free during pregnancy);
Have a facial (very relaxing);
Go swimming – gentle exercise while supported in water is good for you;
Meet friends for lunch;
Visit an exhibition locally;
Arrange to go out one evening;
Plan to do a little cooking: scones and biscuits to offer visitors, soups for quick lunches once the baby is born;
Visit the library and make sure your books are renewed if necessary.
12. Put the champagne in the fridge!

BARE ESSENTIALS FOR THE BABY

Certain items are vital from the beginning. Others can be bought after the baby is born when you may well have a clearer idea of what is needed and what you like.

CLOTHES

It's worth buying several stretch suits to dress the baby in at first. Pretty tops and knitted cardigans are likely to be given as presents, but the basic all-in-one suits can be used for sleeping in and for day wear. Buy half dozen as babies tend to fill their nappies quite often and new parents often find it difficult to prevent said nappies from leaking!

A hat is useful in winter as tiny babies do loose a lot of heat through the head.

Three or four cotton or towelling vests of the kind that have poppers under the crutch are very useful. Because they fit under the baby's bottom, they help hold the nappy on neatly and they don't ride up either. In the summer they can be worn as a cool sun suit and in winter they keep the baby warm under other clothes.

Mittens and booties may be needed for winter babies. You may also need a soft shawl or baby blanket.

See pages 69–75 for more details.

NAPPIES

Even if you plan to use disposables all the time it is worth buying a few towelling nappies. Some babies seem prone to nappy rash and swopping to towelling nappies for a day or two sometimes helps. Often disposable nappies are fine during the day, but as your baby begins (hopefully) to sleep for longer periods at night a towelling nappy may help keep them drier longer.

For more details on nappies see pages 37–44.

If you plan to use towelling nappies you will also need:

Six pairs of plastic pants: tie-on ones are easiest at first. See pages 41–2 for more details.

Disposable nappy liners: available in boxes of 100 and 200. Choose the one-way ones to protect the baby from wetness.

Six safety pins.

Nappy bucket(s). See page 42. Sanitising powder. See pages 42–3.

TOILETRIES

Nappy cream.
Baby lotion (though warm water will do for nappy changes).
Liquid soap for bathing.
Cotton wool.
Tissues.

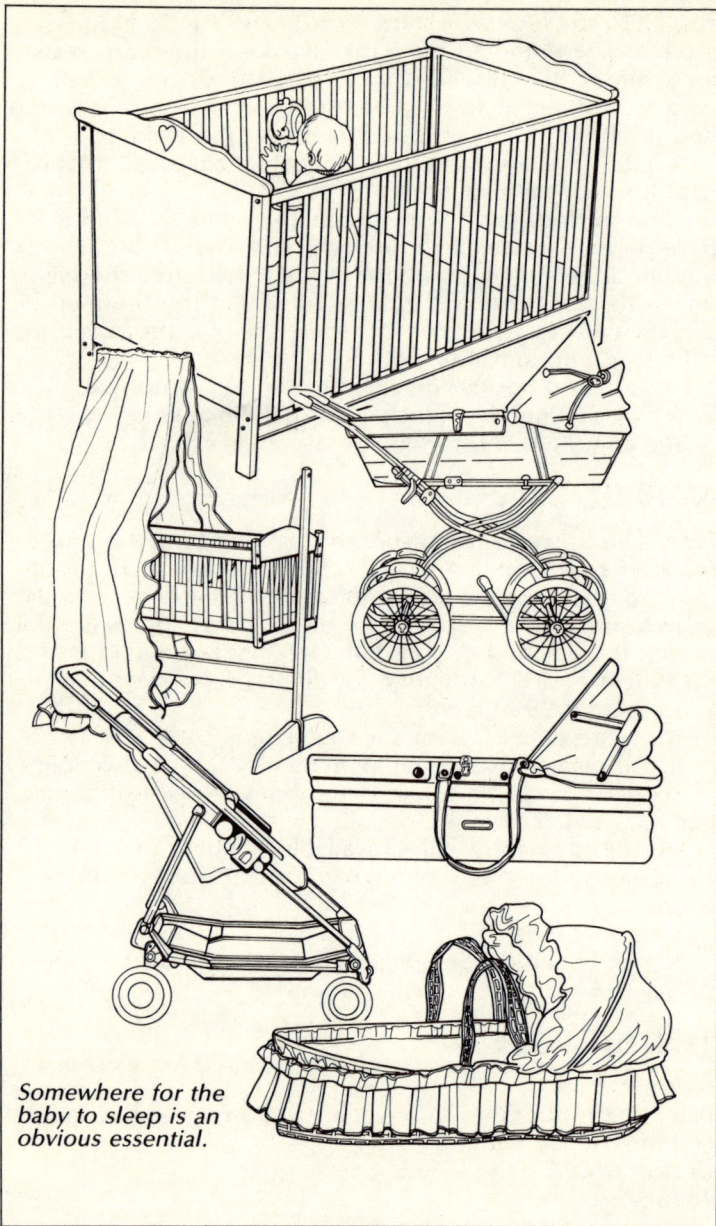

Somewhere for the baby to sleep is an obvious essential.

SOMEWHERE FOR THE BABY TO SLEEP

This obviously another essential. A separate crib or a full-size cot is ideal, or you can use a carrycot or pram top at first, or a Moses basket. For more details on the pros and cons of each see pages 28–31.

SOMETHING TO BATH THE BABY IN

You can use a sink or a large washing up bowl or buy or borrow a baby bath. For more information see pages 61–5.

Put aside or buy a couple of towels for the baby and a flannel or sponge as well.

BOTTLE FEEDING EQUIPMENT

If you are planning to bottle feed, six to eight bottles plus teats and a sterilising unit are essentials too. See pages 51–4.

SOMETHING TO TRANSPORT THE BABY IN

A pram, carrycot and transporter, or a suitable reclining buggy. See pages 77–81 for more information on which type to choose.

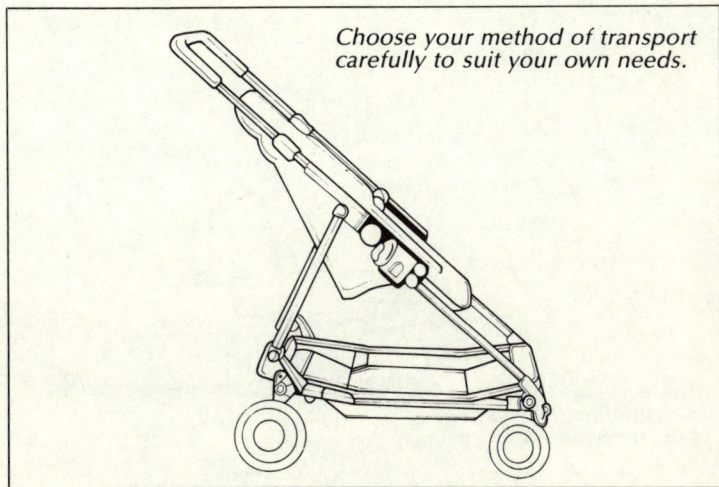

Choose your method of transport carefully to suit your own needs.

USEFUL EXTRAS

You may well choose to buy some of these before your baby is born or they may be given to you as presents. Others can be bought as you need them. Remember that items used for short periods are the ones to borrow, buy secondhand or even hire (see pages 119–124).

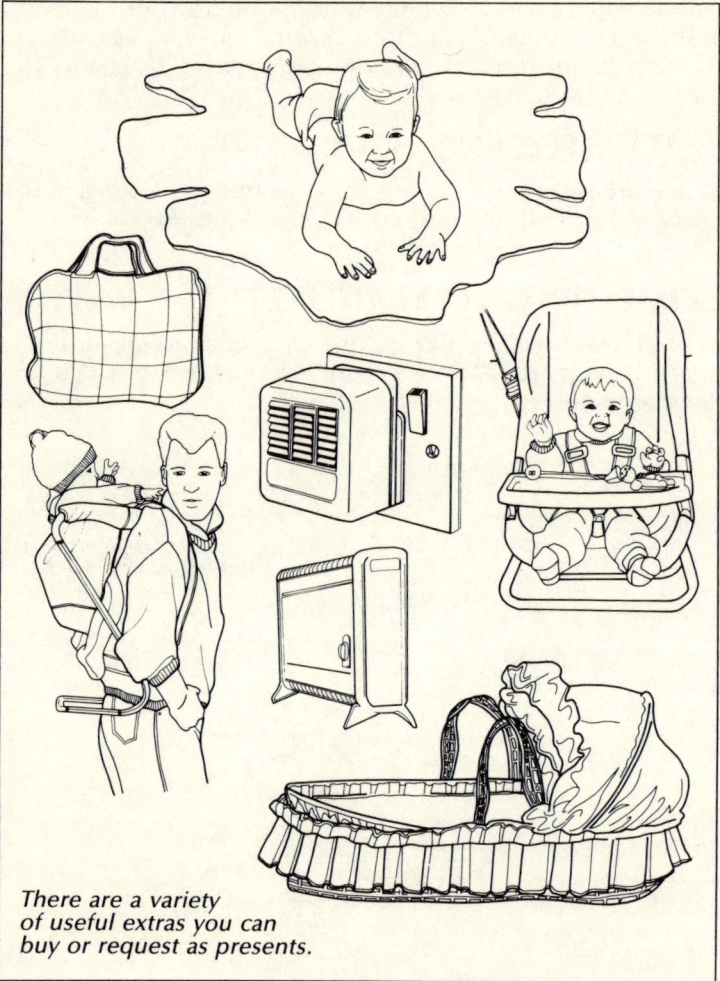

There are a variety of useful extras you can buy or request as presents.

MOSES BASKET OR BABY NEST

These are useful to carry your newborn baby around in.
See page 29.

SLING

Many tiny babies enjoy being carried in a sling. There's a
wide range of types. See pages 86–7 for more details.

BABY SHEEPSKIN

These often help newborns to settle in their cot or pram
and you can take the sheepskin out with you to lie them
on. Page 67 has more details.

NAPPY CHANGING/TRAVELLING BAG

A bag with plenty of pockets and a built-in changing mat
makes it easier to cope with changing nappies when out for
the day. Choose one with shoulder straps so you can carry
the baby and the bag safely. Make sure the outside will
wipe clean or that the whole bag is washable. Pretty fabric
bags are available as kits to sew or there's a wide range of
suitable bags on the market. Remember as babies get older
you have to carry more: cups, dishes, bibs, changes of
clothes, favourite toys, etc. so allow plenty of space in the
bag you choose.

BOUNCING CHAIR

See pages 89–90.

HEATER

A heater for the baby's room is useful, especially if your
baby will be born in the winter. Tiny babies cannot control
their own body temperature properly. External heating is
vital at first. Aim to have the room at around
16–18°C/60–65°F overnight at first. You may find you need
extra heating during the day as well.

Remember very cold babies don't cry, it wastes their
energy. Feel behind the baby's neck, just under his clothes
(where the label usually is), to check body temperature.
Hands and feet often feel quite cold when the rest of the
body is actually warm.

Overheating is also a problem as babies cannot cool themselves down very well either! A room thermometer is quite useful so you can keep the temperature about right.

COT

A cot, a mattress with a ventilated top section, cot sheets, blankets, etc. If you start off with a crib you can often delay buying a cot for three to four months until the baby outgrows the crib. See page 29.

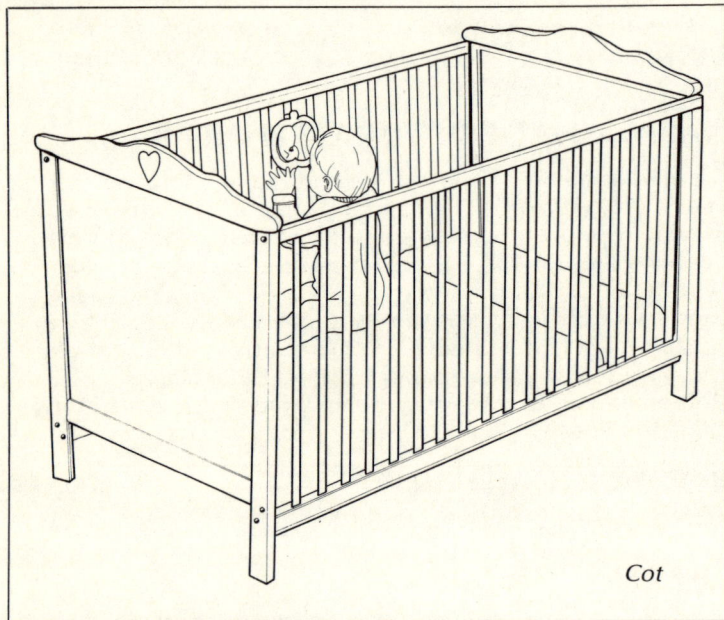

Cot

CAR SAFETY RESTRAINTS

These are essential to fix the carry cot unless you have a special baby seat to be used with an adult seat belt. See pages 82–4.

BABY ALARM

These are especially useful if the baby's room is a long way from your bedroom or you are unlikely to hear the baby downstairs. See pages 35–6.

PADDED CHANGING MAT

These have a wipe-clean finish, and can be used on the floor, on a special dresser or in a cot. See page 37.

PERSONAL CHECKLISTS

HOSPITAL BAG FOR MOTHER IN LABOUR

- [ ] Nightdress
- [ ] Natural sponge
- [ ] Lip salve
- [ ] Focus object
- [ ] Hairbrush
- [ ] Slides or ribbon
- [ ] Cassette tapes and recorder
- [ ] Massage oil or baby lotion
- [ ] Flannel
- [ ] Toothbrush
- [ ] Toothpaste
- [ ] Hot water bottle and cover
- [ ] Mirror

GENERAL BAG FOR HOSPITAL

- [ ] Nightdress
- [ ] Dressing gown
- [ ] Slippers
- [ ] Feeding bras
- [ ] Nipple cream
- [ ] Soap
- [ ] Flannel
- [ ] Toothbrush
- [ ] Toothpaste
- [ ] Large and small towels
- [ ] Hairbrush
- [ ] Shampoo
- [ ] Deodorant
- [ ] Make-up
- [ ] Perfume
- [ ] Salt
- [ ] Books or magazines
- [ ] Writing paper and envelopes
- [ ] Pen
- [ ] Stamps

☐	Address book
☐	Birth announcement cards
☐	Coins for telephone
☐	Hair dryer or curling tongs
☐	Sanitary towels and pants

HOSPITAL BAG FOR BABY

☐	Disposable nappies
☐	Tissues
☐	Cotton wool
☐	Liquid soap
☐	Petroleum jelly
☐	Clothes to wear home

HOSPITAL BAG FOR FATHER/LABOUR PARTNER

☐	Flask of tea/coffee/cold drinks.
☐	Snackfoods
☐	Telephone numbers
☐	Change for the telephone
☐	Camera and film
☐	Cotton short-sleeved T-shirt
☐	Note pad and pencil

BARE ESSENTIALS FOR THE BABY

Clothes

- [ ] 6 stretch suits
- [ ] Hat
- [ ] 4 button-under vests
- [ ] Mittens
- [ ] Booties
- [ ] Shawl

Nappies

- [ ] 24 nappies (or 60 disposables)
- [ ] 6 pairs plastic pants
- [ ] Disposable nappy liners
- [ ] 6 safety pins
- [ ] Nappy bucket
- [ ] Sanitising powder

Toiletries

- [ ] Nappy cream
- [ ] Baby lotion
- [ ] Liquid soap
- [ ] Cotton wool
- [ ] Tissues

Miscellaneous

- [ ] Cot, crib or carrycot
- [ ] Bath
- [ ] Pram, carrycot and transporter or buggy

Bottle Feeding Equipment

- [ ] Formula milk
- [ ] 6–8 bottles
- [ ] Teats
- [ ] Sterilising unit

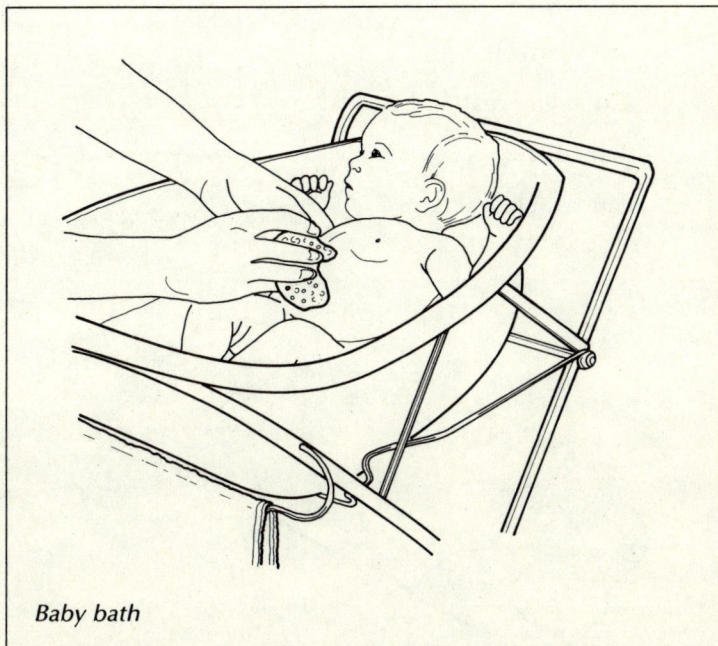

Baby bath

USEFUL EXTRAS

- [ ] Moses basket
- [ ] Baby nest
- [ ] Sling
- [ ] Baby sheepskin
- [ ] Nappy changing/travelling bag
- [ ] Bouncing chair
- [ ] Heater
- [ ] Cot
- [ ] Cot mattress
- [ ] Cot sheets
- [ ] Cot blankets
- [ ] Car safety restraints
- [ ] Baby alarm
- [ ] Padded changing mat

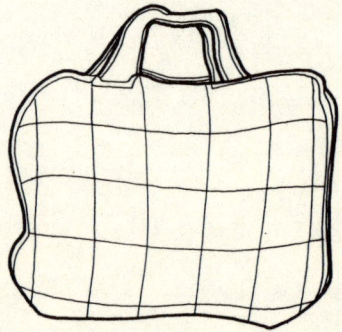

Nappy changing bag

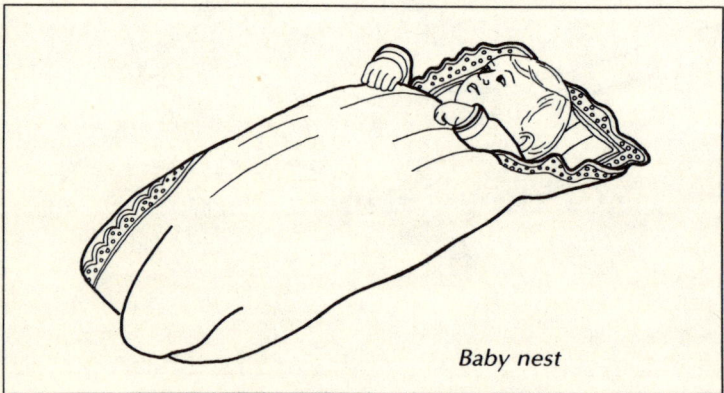

Baby nest

2 NEW BABIES

This chapter concentrates on the basics of caring for your baby with plenty of tips on equipment to choose, plus shortcuts and hints from experienced mums on coping with your baby.

SLEEPING
SOMEWHERE TO SLEEP

The choice here is between a crib, carrycot or Moses basket and stand for the first few months, and then a cot.

CRIBS

Cribs look lovely, and you may have a family heirloom you want to use, otherwise it is a good idea to try to borrow

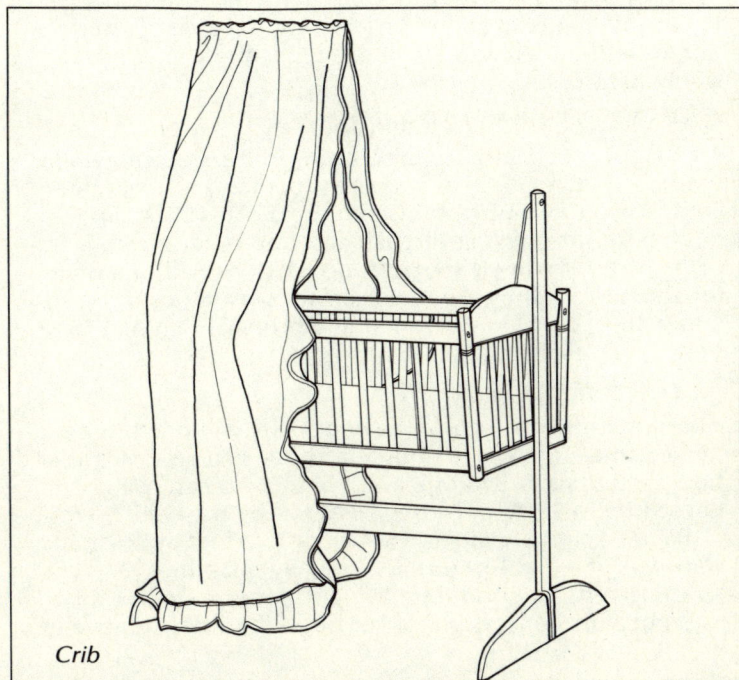

Crib

one. They are only used for the first six months at most so try not to be tempted into spending too much on one. Check how stable the crib is, and if there are any rough points that may catch on your clothes as you pass, causing you to pull it over.

MOSES BASKETS

Moses baskets are useful to carry the baby around in as well as to sleep in. Check how the handles are fixed to the basket; those woven in underneath rather than fixed to the top of the basket spread the load and will wear better. Some Moses baskets have fabric sun hoods.

Stands are available with some Moses baskets to turn the basket into a crib. These are useful to lift the basket off the floor and keep it out of draughts if you plan to let the baby sleep in it overnight.

If you want to line a crib or basket yourself, choose a quilted cotton fabric for warmth and comfort. Quilted fabrics have the advantage of not falling in on top of the baby. Even so it is wise to tie the lining on at the handle. Reversible material allows you to ring the changes and minimise the washing. Some are available with vented safety mattresses.

CARRYCOTS AND STANDS

A carrycot on a stand can also be used for sleeping while the baby is tiny. Plastic-lined carrycots tend to feel rather cold, so you may want to use an extra blanket. Again they double up for carrying the baby around in, and with a set of transporter wheels they can be used instead of a pram for short trips. They are however not very well sprung so if you plan to do plenty of walking a proper pram may be a better buy. (See pages 77–81.)

COTS AND COT BEDS

At around four to six months your baby will need to be moved to a large cot. Be guided by his size and weight and how mobile he is. Don't leave a baby who can roll or pull himself up in a crib or Moses basket as he may well tip it up.

Babies generally move from a cot to a bed at any stage between one and three years. Usually once they start trying to climb out is a good time to consider introducing a bed.

Some cots convert into a cot bed. The sides remove and

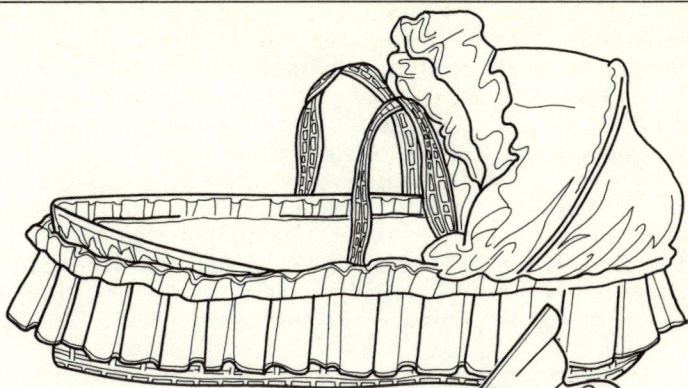

Moses basket

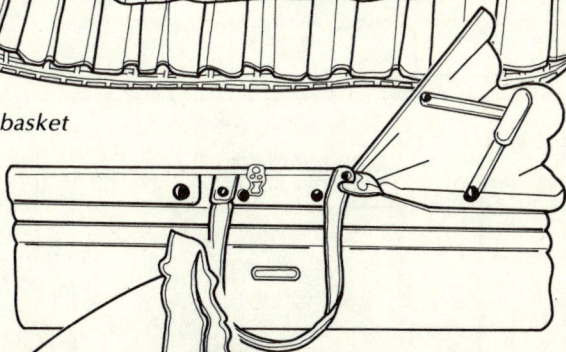

Carrycot

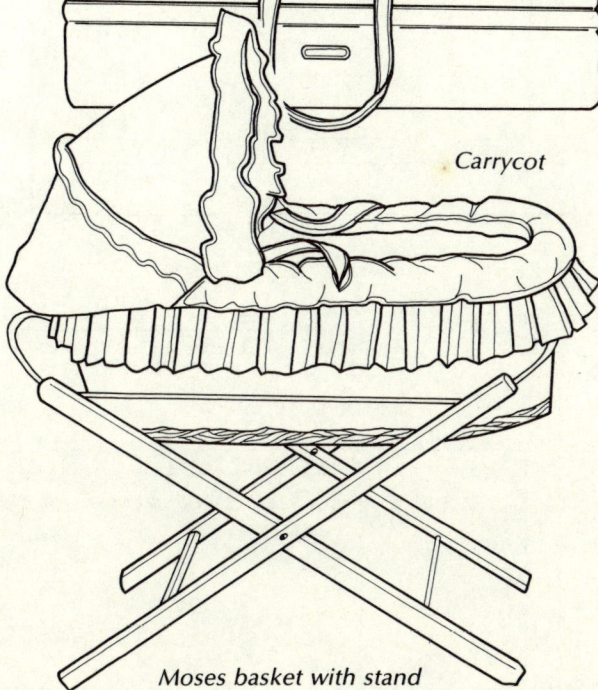

Moses basket with stand

the base can be set very low making the transition from cot to bed easier. These are smaller than an ordinary bed though, so expect to move the baby into a larger bed by the time he is four to five. If you do opt for a cot bed, remember it will be in use for longer than a cot so won't be available as a cot for a second child.

Cots are covered by a British Standard which specifies the gap between the bars. Drop sides are useful to make it easier to lift the baby in and out. Some cots can have the base and mattress at three different heights, so you can move the base down as the baby gets older. If you choose one of these, don't leave it too late before moving the base down.

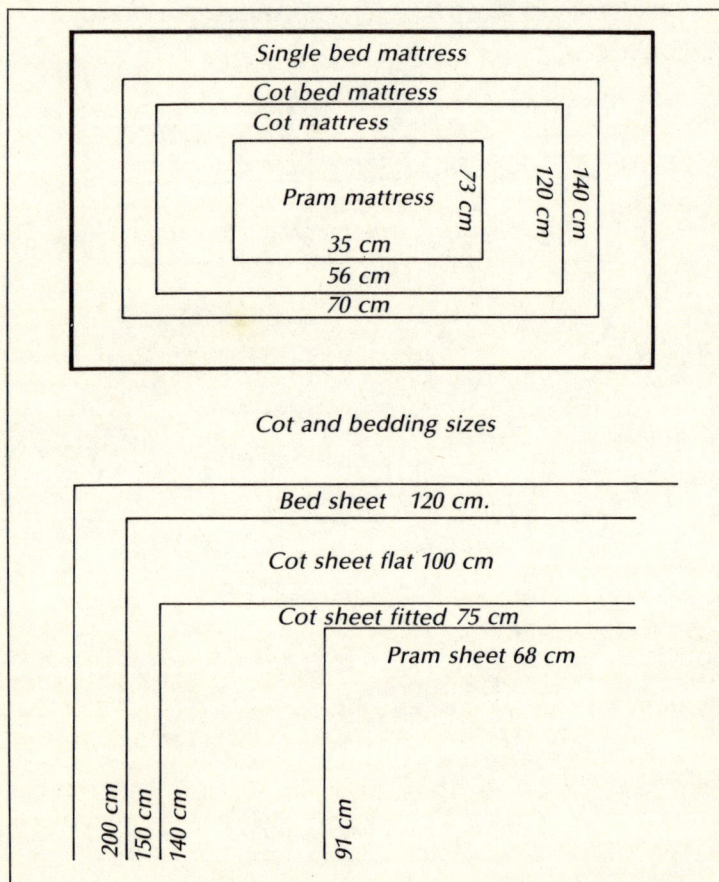

Single bed mattress
Cot bed mattress
Cot mattress
Pram mattress
73 cm
120 cm
140 cm
35 cm
56 cm
70 cm

Cot and bedding sizes

Bed sheet   120 cm.
Cot sheet flat 100 cm
Cot sheet fitted 75 cm
Pram sheet 68 cm
200 cm
150 cm
140 cm
91 cm

MATTRESSES AND BEDDING

MATTRESSES

Vented cot mattresses, sometimes called 'safety mattresses', have small holes punched in the top. Tiny babies cannot turn their heads, so if they vomit they may inhale it. Vented mattresses prevent the vomit pooling, and allow the baby to continue breathing.

Foam vented mattresses are usually considered the best for babies. They give good support and don't often cause allergies.

Most cot mattresses have a waterproof cover. Waterproof sheets are available for uncovered mattresses but tend to become dislodged as the baby moves around.

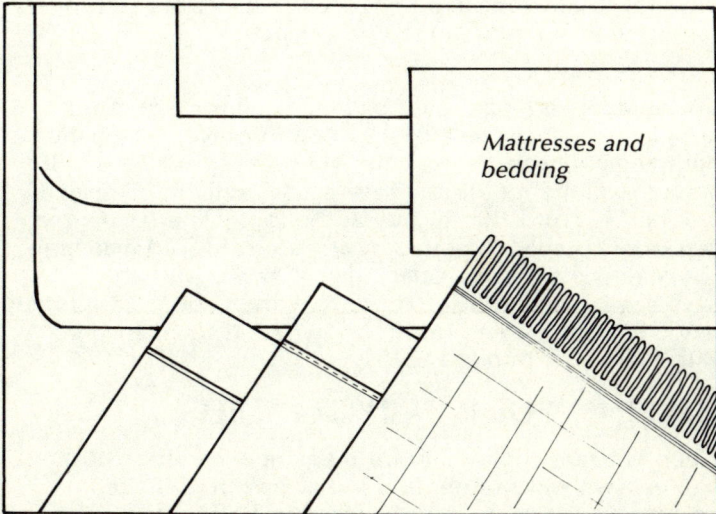

Mattresses and bedding

PILLOWS

Babies under twelve months should not have a pillow. They don't miss pillows and will happily sleep on flat mattresses. If you really need to raise the mattress, (for instance if your baby has a cold and is snuffly) put a small pillow or folded blanket under the mattress so the baby sleeps on a slight slope, or raise the cot by standing the front legs on a piece of wood.

QUILTS

Quilts are useful for slightly older babies. However, under six months a baby cannot wriggle out from under the quilt if he gets too hot. This, combined with the fact that most babies seem to like being well tucked in, means that blankets are a better buy for the first six months. Cut costs by buying blankets to fit a full-sized cot and use them doubled in a crib or pram. Cellular blankets are light and warm and will also double up as a shawl.

SHEETS

Flanellette sheets are warm and soft and wash well. Fitted cot sheets are available in both cotton and polyester mixtures and in stretch terry toweling. These make a cot quicker to change, and help prevent the baby untucking the sheets. Buy four to six sheets to begin with. Flat sheets can be used doubled up in cribs or prams.

COT BUMPERS

Cot bumpers are patterned padded sections that stand upright around the side of the cot and prevent the baby bumping his head on the bars. They look pretty and help keep the draught out too. They usually only fit half-way around the cot. Either fit one at the top of the cot, or buy two to fit completely round. Many are sold with matching cot covers and sheets. Check that they are washable or have a wipe-clean finish. Those that are made from quilted fabric have a tendency to droop, whereas foam covered with fabric stay in place better.

HELPING YOUR BABY TO SLEEP

Sleep is a rare commodity for many new parents. Most babies have wakeful periods and sleepy periods, but it often takes weeks or months for your baby's sleeping cycle to become synchronised with yours. Often babies go on needing night feeds for much longer than parents expect.

There seem to be three elements involved in comforting a crying baby and helping them to sleep: touch, sound and movement. Rocking your baby in your arms and singing to him combines all three of these and is often comforting to parents too. However, if you tire of this and need a break try one or more of the following ideas.

SWADDLING

Swaddling helps some tiny babies feel secure and settled. Wrap your baby firmly in a light blanket, with his arms folded against his body and lie him in his cot or pram on his side. You may need to use a small folded blanket or nappy against his back to prevent him rolling over.

SHEEPSKINS

Special washable baby sheepskins are useful too. They were originally used in some premature baby units and are now widely available. It seems the warmth and tactile stimulation helps some babies to settle. For best results start using it early, within the first few weeks.

CUDDLIES

A cuddly is a special toy or a silky cloth for the baby to cuddle, and this often helps him to settle to sleep. Be prepared for this cuddly to become a vital part of your baby's life, though. You may be able to have a spare, or cut a cuddle cloth in half just in case the original becomes lost.

NOISE

Noise helps some babies to sleep. Often constant background noise, like the vacuum cleaner or the washing machine in use, will help a tiny baby drift off to sleep. If you tire of constantly doing the vacuuming to persuade the baby to settle down you can buy a tape of 'white noise' which generally has the same effect. Also available is a tape of 'womb music' which plays the soporific gurgles and rhythmic heart beat sounds the baby used to hear *in utero*. Both these tapes should be started within the first ten weeks to be effective.

ROCKING

Rocking a baby up and down can help too. Put the baby in the pram and take him for a walk, or go for a car ride if desperate. An automatic pram rocker is available too. It hooks on the pram handle and uses a revolving weight to rock the pram up and down. Also available is a hammock that can be tied onto a full-size cot. It has a synthetic sheepskin lining and a battery-operated heart beat sound so that the baby is gently rocked to sleep. A net fixed to a large spring can be bought to hold a carry cot or Moses basket. This can be gently rocked up and down to settle the baby.

A rocking chair is a very comfortable way of sitting rocking your baby and many babies settle if they are carried close to your body in a sling.

ROUTINE

Routine begins to matter at around eight to ten weeks. It's worth establishing a regular bedtime as soon as possible. Often a bath before bed tires the baby out and makes him feel warm and sleepy. Follow with a cuddle and a feed and then put the baby in his crib or cot. You may well have to pick him up several times during the evening and night to feed him, but try to keep night feeds low-key affairs. Use a small lamp or a dimmer switch and feed and change the baby quietly. As your baby grows you may find he is woken by the light mornings. A thick blind or a curtain over the window may keep the light out and gain you a few extra hours sleep.

BABY ALARMS

An alarm means that you can put your baby to sleep in the cot and still be able to eavesdrop on him from time to time. Traditionally they have required a wire to connect the alarm and speaker, but the new 'plug in' models do away with this. They use the household wiring system to convey sounds and are ideal to use when staying with friends and grandparents. Some need to be used on the same ring main and others simply need the wiring to all sockets to run back to the same fuse box and meter. Do check when buying them, as some large houses have separate ring circuits for the upstairs and downstairs.

If you choose a wired model ensure there is sufficient wire to reach from the baby's room to the living room and also try to arrange it so the wire does not have to be folded or looped as this can cause crackling.

Voice activated models turn themselves on if the baby begins to make a noise, instead of remaining on all the time. This saves on batteries and avoids the temptation to listen all the time.

Two-way alarms allow you to talk to the baby, although the quality of reception varies. Often with older children just hearing your voice helps them to settle down again.

This type can often be used as intercoms later. Some of the more sophisticated baby alarms have a volume control on both the baby's end and on the speaker end. This is useful as it allows you to set the sending alarm according to how loudly your baby breathes and snores when he is asleep and to make allowances for having to position the alarm some way from the baby's cot. A volume control on the receiving end ensures you will hear even if the television or radio is on.

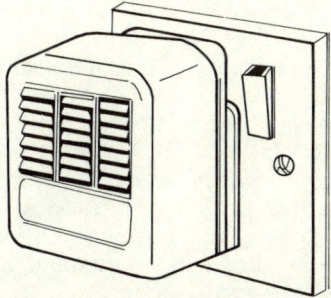

Plug-in alarm

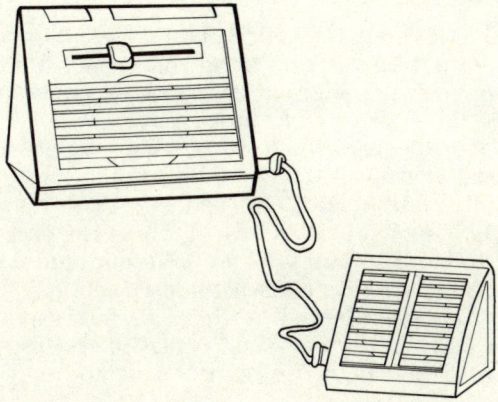

Two-way alarm

TIPS ON GETTING YOUR BABY TO SLEEP

1. Make sure the baby is not hungry or thirsty.
2. Make sure he is comfortable — not too warm or cold, not wet or dirty.
3. Is the light okay? A bright light may be annoying, or complete darkness frightening.
4. Is it too noisy or too quiet?
5. Is the baby in his favourite sleeping position?
6. If the baby has a special toy or blanket to sleep with, make sure you always give it to them. And also keep a spare one for emergencies.
7. Rocking or gentle movement helps some children to go to sleep.
8. Some babies like to watch a mobile or similar toy while they are going to sleep.
9. Some babies enjoy a comfort suck from breast or bottle before they go to sleep.
10. Establish a bedtime routine as early as practical and stick to it. Make it enjoyable but relaxing.
11. Even very small babies may enjoy a bedtime story and a cuddle long before they can understand what you are reading. It gives you a chance to re-read some of your own favourite children's books.

NAPPIES

The average baby gets through 3,500 to 4,500 nappy changes during the two years or so they need them. New parents soon become adept at changing nappies; after all it needs to be done six to eight times a day at first!

It's well worth organising a nappy changing area in the baby's room. A firm worktop or the top of a chest of drawers at the right height, with space to store nappies, plastic pants, creams, pins etc. is all that is needed. Keep everything to hand so you will never be tempted to leave the baby on the worktop even for a few seconds. Alternatively keep all the nappy changing items in a basket and move it around as necessary. A plastic-covered padded changing mat is useful as it is comfortable and easy to wipe clean.

The basic choice is between disposables and terry nappies. In practice many parents find they use a combination of the two.

DISPOSABLE NAPPIES

Disposables are certainly convenient and quick to use. They are ideal when travelling. For anyone with limited laundry facilities they save the hard work of washing and drying nappies, too. They are, of course, a regular expense. However the true cost of washing and drying terry nappies will amount to the same sort of figure (including detergent, hot water, running a washing machine, tumble drying and plastic pants and nappy liners).

Disposables used to leak a great deal, but elasticated legs have overcome this problem. Resealable tapes have helped improve the problem of tapes not sticking, and made it easier to get the nappy to fit the baby; if the nappy falls down when you stand him up at least you can undo it and re-stick the tapes!

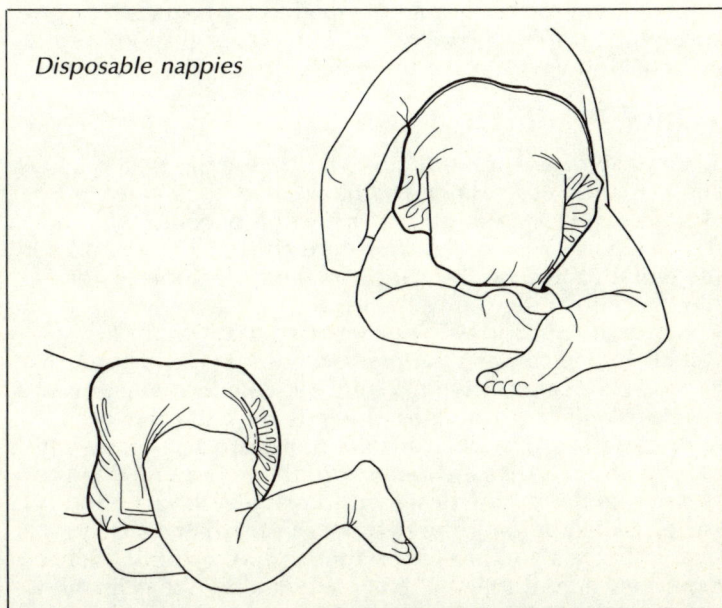

Disposable nappies

I tested a whole range of disposable nappies for *Mother* magazine. We used around 2,500 nappies on 40 babies of different sexes and ages. Each family was given a selection of nappies in unmarked bags, so they did not know which brand they were using (obviously some guessed, but they were only right about half the time).

Our general results showed that nappies with elasticated legs and resealable tapes were the most popular and most effective. Interestingly, we also found that nappies varied in shape and size considerably, so as your baby grows and changes from a slim newborn baby to a six-month-old with a distinct tummy you may find you have to change brands to find one that fits.

Used disposables should not be flushed down the toilet. Seal in a plastic bag and place in the dustbin. Some parents like to use a disposable liner so that the worst of the soiling can be flushed down the loo. Scented bags are available to use to throw away disposables. They are expensive, but useful when travelling or visiting.

Disposable nappies are bulky to store, but very large packs are often the cheapest way to buy them. Nappy delivery services are usually quite competitive, so check prices. Generous grandparents might be persuaded to give a month's supply of nappies delivered to your door as a present to help you over the hard work of the first weeks.

TERRY NAPPIES

Terry nappies are soft and absorbent. Buy the best quality you can afford since they will be washed constantly for around two years and cheap ones soon become thin and frayed. Disposable nappy liners are cheap to buy and keep the worst soiling off the nappy, making cleaning easier. Always choose the one-way liners.

Buy 24 terry nappies. They will last about four days so will allow you to wash nappies every other day. Most people choose plain white ones, but coloured versions are now available, with pink or blue edging. Extra thick night-time nappies are available. Some are also made with a small amount of elastic material in them to allow them to stetch slightly. This is designed to make getting a good fit easier. In fact folding the nappy to fit the baby is quite a knack. There's a choice of methods of folding but to the expectant parent they all tend to look a bit like origami!

Triangular-shaped nappies with a padded central section are also made. They do give a very neat fit, but are nowhere near as absorbent as a full-size terry nappy which, once folded, has several layers of towelling to absorb the wetness.

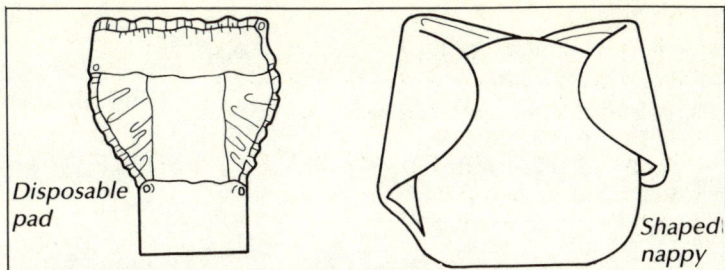

Disposable pad

Shaped nappy

Always remember to keep your hand between the pin and the baby when securing terry nappies.

FOLDING NAPPIES

CHINESE FOLD

This fold makes the smallest and neatest nappy so it is ideal for tiny babies. It also has the advantage of plenty of thickness where it is needed.

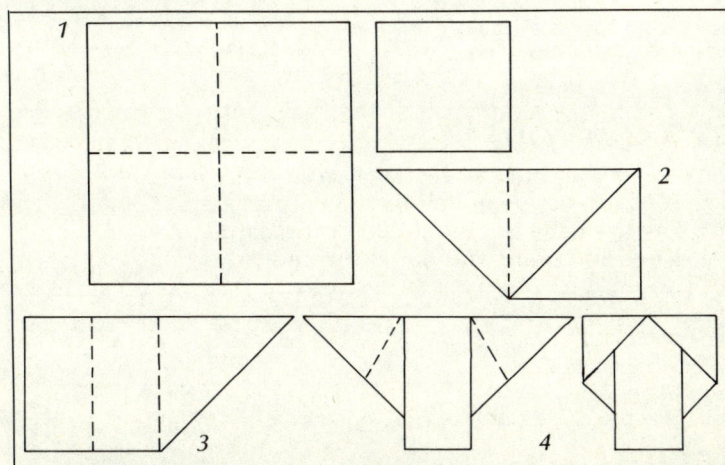

1. Fold the nappy into quarters.
2. Take the top corner and pull it horizontally to make a triangle.
3. Turn the nappy over so that triangle is underneath. Fold the top section into three so it sits in the middle of the triangle.
4. Fold the top and sides into the middle over the baby and pin in the centre.

KITE FOLD

This is the simplest and most common fold.
1. Fold in two sides to meet in the middle.
2. Fold the top down to make a kite shape.
3. Fold the point inside.
4. Fold the sides and bottom over the baby and secure with one or two pins.

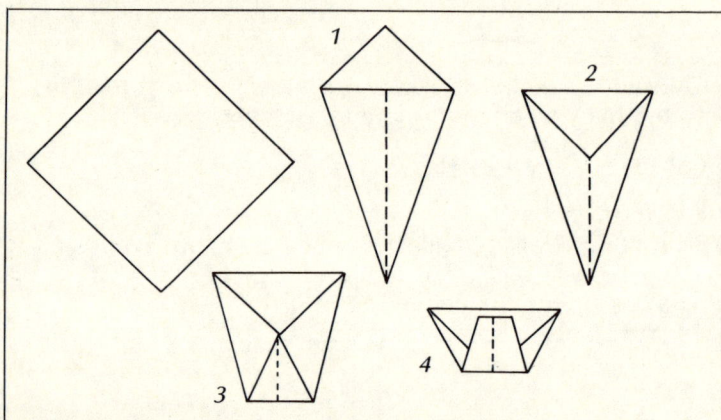

TRIANGLE FOLD

This is simple, but can be baggy round the legs.
1. Fold the nappy in half to form a triangle.
2. Lay the baby in the middle of the nappy. Fold in the sides and point and pin at the centre.

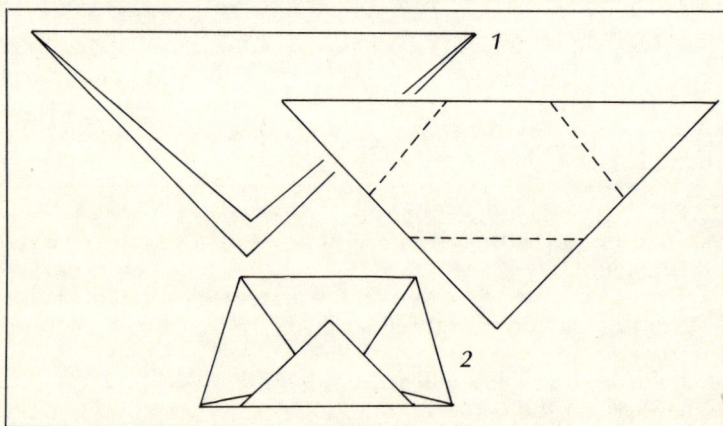

NAPPY LINERS

These help keep the moisture away from the baby's skin and catch the worst of the soiling, leaving the nappy cleaner than it would be.

Disposable ones are available as straightforward liners, or one-way liners. The latter are slightly more expensive but very effective. They pass the moisture through into the terry nappy but don't let it back to sit against the baby's skin.

Fabric liners are useful for babies with very delicate skins (when the muslin type can be used inside a terry nappy) and some have the same one-way action as disposable one-way liners. They are useful to use at night or if your baby has a nappy rash.

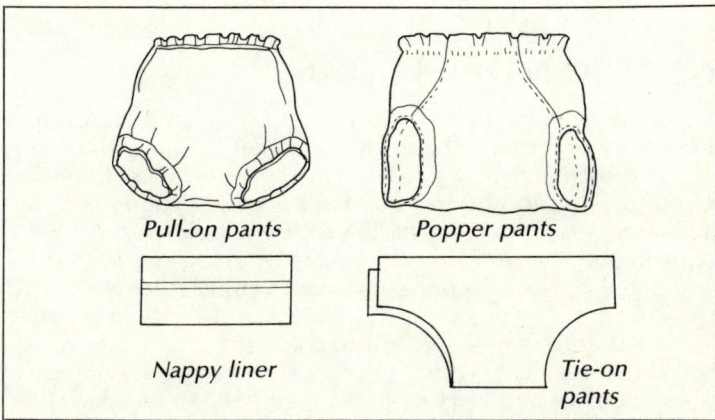

Pull-on pants   Popper pants

Nappy liner   Tie-on
                       pants

PLASTIC PANTS

All-in-one disposable nappies have the plastic pants built in. Terry nappies need a pair of plastic pants on top. It can be difficult to get ordinary plastic pants to fit newborn babies. Tie-on pants are a useful idea. They come in packs of five or ten and are cheap to buy, as they are simply shaped flat sheets of plastic. They tie on top of the nappy and can be adjusted to fit the baby.

As the baby grows pull-on pants and popper pants become more practical. In a test of over 20 brands of plastic pants we found the popper pants useful when dealing with really mucky nappies as they could be undone rather than slid down the baby's legs.

Many brands of plastic pants can only be handwashed, which is a great disadvantage and not very hygienic. After a few washes many become stiff and uncomfortable for the baby. Some more expensive brands can be machine washed and will remain soft and supple for a long time. So either buy cheap ones and then throw them away after a few weeks, or choose the more expensive ones and wash them in the machine. Avoid putting them in sanitising solution as they will discolour and become stiff and cracked very quickly.

If you want babies to look pretty under summer dresses, some plastic pants have a fabric outer. They vary from nylon lacy ones to real cotton broderie anglais. These are attractive and nice to have when you want to dress your baby up. They are more expensive than the plain ones but you are likely to need less of them.

GETTING NAPPIES CLEAN

Sluice off the worst of the soiling in the toilet. Hold on to the nappy firmly and then pull the chain so the rush of water does the cleaning for you. Then either soak them in sanitising solution or boil them. Sanitising solution is in fact a bleach. It will shorten the life of the nappies but is very convenient. Be careful not to splash your clothes with it and avoid soaking coloured or wool baby clothes in it. You can substitute ordinary bleach. Bleaches do vary in strength but a half to one egg cup full to one bucket of water is usually about right. However, nappy sanitising solution is not expensive and lasts quite a long time.

If you plan to boil nappies you will need a large old saucepan and a pair of tongs. Deal with a few nappies at a time. Mix a little washing powder with the water, bring to the boil on the cooker and boil for five minutes. Stir with the tongs during this time. Then remove the nappies and rinse and dry.

Two nappy buckets make life easier since each will hold six to eight nappies: an average day's needs. Two day's needs (12 to 16 nappies) makes an automatic washing machine load. So every other day you can drain and rinse the nappies and wash them in a long hot wash. Rinsing is important as the sanitising solution can affect the door seals on a washing machine. A long hot wash will get the nappies clean. In theory using sanitising solution means that you can just rinse the nappies, but in practice this tends to leave the nappies discoloured.

Fabric conditioner will make the nappies fluffy, but occasionally babies are sensitive to it. Try it and see: if your baby develops a rash over the area the nappy comes into contact with, and not just where he is wet it may be the fabric conditioner. Alternatively it could be that the nappies are not rinsed well enough and there are still traces of detergent in them.

Whenever possible dry nappies out on the line. A good blow in the fresh air will soften them, the sunshine will help bleach out any remaining stains and kill some bacteria which may cause nappy rash.

NAPPY RASH

This is really very common, but it's uncomfortable for the baby and worrying for the parents. Nip it in the bud by changing nappies frequently and allowing the baby to spend some time each day without his nappy on. Tiny babies can be laid on towels or on the changing mat to have a kick for ten minutes or so. Mobile babies are more difficult. In summer, a play in the garden without his nappy on helps. In winter you just have to keep your fingers crossed and be nearby with a cloth to mop up any accidents.

Plastic pants which keep the baby's bottom warm and moist are partly to blame, so putting on a terry nappy but not plastic pants or clothes on top often helps. At least that way you know when he is wet!

Changing the type of nappy sometimes helps too; from disposables to terries and vice versa.

There's a wide range of creams for nappy rash to choose from. The homoeopathic ones can help and so too can a cream based on wool fat. Your chemist will advise which to try. You can sometimes borrow a cream from a friend to see if it has any effect before you buy a whole pot.

If the nappy rash persists, or it is severe enough to make the baby cry each time he urinates, then do consult your doctor. There are creams available on prescription which can help, and indeed some nappy rashes may not be a simple rash but have a specific cause, such as thrush.

Avoid using mineral-based oils on a baby with a bottom

that is beginning to look a bit sore as it can dry the skin. As urine is acidic, washing the baby's skin in warm water plus just a little bicarbonate of soda dissolved in it, sometimes makes the baby more comfortable. Allow it to dry completely before putting on the cream. Overnight, spread his bottom and the whole affected area with a thick layer of cream to help the skin heal and to keep him comfortable.

TEN QUICK TIPS ON NAPPIES

1. Fold terry nappies in to the right shape and stack near the changing mat. Then you won't be attempting to fold the nappy and hold on to a wriggling baby.
2. If you don't have a chest of drawers to change the baby on put the changing mat in the cot (with the side down) and change the baby there.
3. Choose nappy buckets with a holder in the lid for an air freshener block. Some also have 'strainers' to allow the water to be drained off without the nappies slipping out too.
4. Once your baby is mobile, stand nappy buckets in the bath to prevent him tipping them over as he pulls himself up on them.
5. Disposables often leak when babies are totally breast fed (the stools of breast-fed babies are mustardy yellow and quite liquid). Overcome this by using tie-on plastic pants on top.
6. At night use double terry nappies for more absorbency. Put two together flat then fold as usual. An insert disposable nappy pad can also be used either inside a terry nappy or inside an all-in-one disposable.
7. Save plastic bags from supermarket shopping for sealing used disposable nappies in. Store them safely in a high cupboard or shelf.
8. Keep a terry nappy or old towel by the changing mat to wipe your hands on after putting cream on the baby's bottom. Greasy fingers will prevent the sticky tabs on disposables sticking.
9. If tabs will not stick, secure with a length of plaster. It holds better than ordinary sticky tape.
10. Make sure you put a disposable nappy on properly. Unfold the plastic edges around the gathered leg piece so they stick out once the nappy is on. Tuck in the extra plastic at the waist. Avoid tucking vests in to the nappy as the dampness will seep up the vest.

FEEDING YOUR BABY

How you feed your baby is entirely up to you. Breast feeding is undoubtedly the best for your baby. It supplies antibodies which give your baby protection against some infections. It's perfectly suited for your baby, the sucking action of a breast-fed baby helps the jaw to develop and it also ensures that the new mother has to sit down and rest at regular intervals while feeding! It helps the uterus contract after the birth, too. Many women find they enjoy breast feeding their babies once the process is well established. It's also easy and convenient.

Some women and their partners find it embarrassing. Others find that problems in the early days make it too daunting to continue. Bottle feeding is a useful option. All mothers have the choice of doing what suits them best.

BREAST FEEDING

A good nursing bra can go a long way towards making the first few days of breast feeding more comfortable. During the last few weeks of pregnancy and the first few days after your baby is born your breasts contain colostrum. This is a creamy colour and texture, and although there is not a great deal of it, it is very valuable to your baby. At around

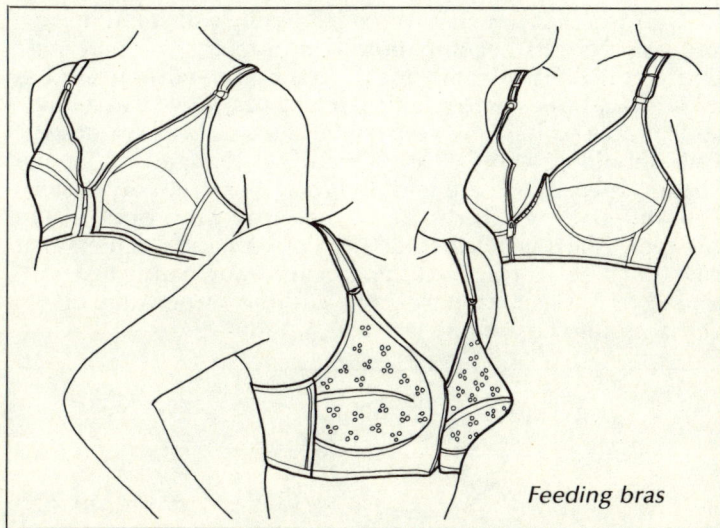

Feeding bras

day three to four after the birth, your breasts begin to make milk in quantity. Often your breasts feel very full and hard at this stage and increase in size quite dramatically. A supportive bra, preferably in cotton, is vital at this stage. Choose one with non-elasticated straps and a generous width of material on the sides. It needs to be adjustable to cope with both the increase in size as your milk comes in and the decrease as your milk settles down. Drop flap bras can be uncomfortable in the early days and if they cut into the breast the pressure can block the milk ducts. Opt for a front opening bra if possible. Most have a strap underneath the cups so the other side of the bra will remain done up while feeding.

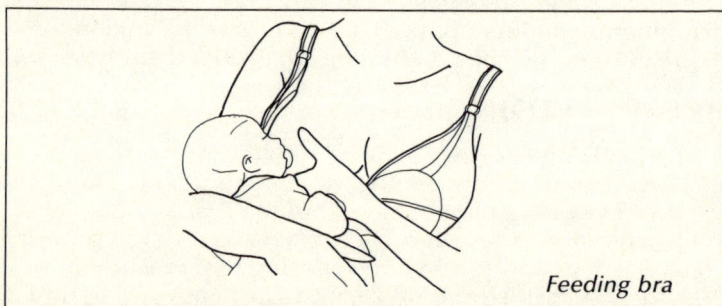

Feeding bra

After the first few days the milk supply will settle down and your breasts become more comfortable. You may still find you leak milk from your breasts and need to use breast pads. Avoid ones with plastic backings as these can allow your nipple to become very wet and encourage soreness. Pads should absorb excess milk and be changed frequently. Shaped breast pads are a little thicker but quite expensive. Reusable pads which can be washed may work out cheaper. Alternatives include old cotton handkerchiefs that have become soft with washing or one-way nappy liners folded to fit. Even sanitary pads, cut into three will work and are quite absorbent.

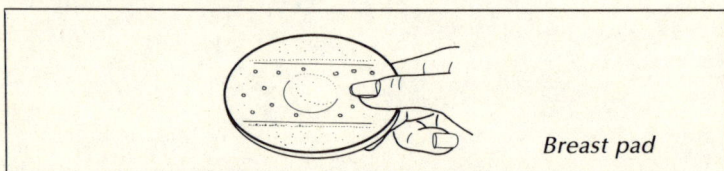

Breast pad

SORENESS

Soreness is common in the first few days of breast feeding. After all nipples are usually quite sensitive! Making sure your baby is in a good position and has taken most of the areola (the dark area around the nipple) into his mouth will help. The nipple needs to be well into his mouth so that he can squeeze with his lips and gums to get the milk. It's a completely different action to sucking from a teat. Your midwife will help you at first, and ensure the baby is properly 'fixed' or 'latched on'. You may find changing the position the baby feeds in helps to cope with soreness. Ask your midwife to help you try feeding the baby lying down or with his feet tucked under your arm, lying on a pillow.

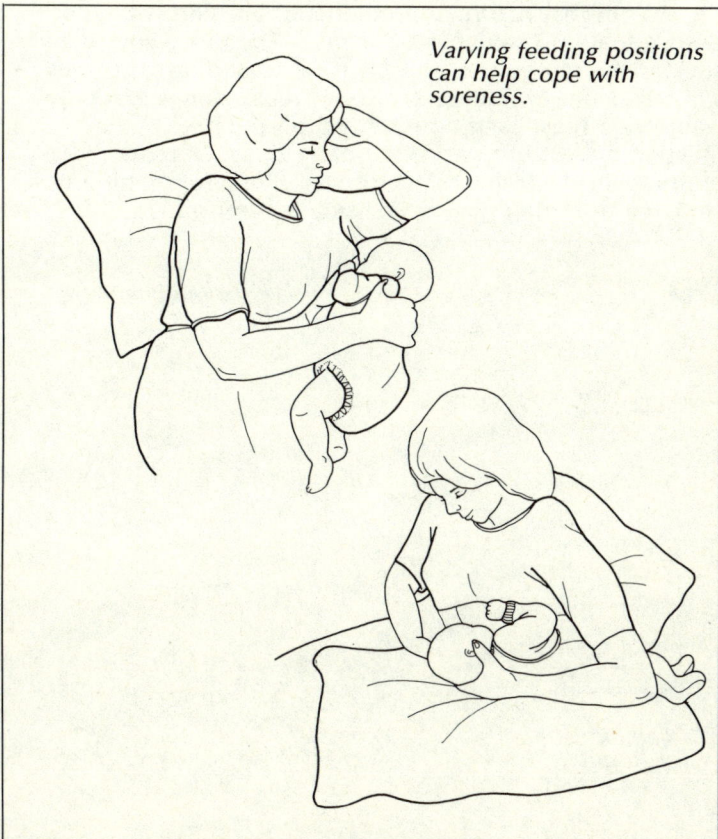

Varying feeding positions can help cope with soreness.

Creams can help with soreness too. Homoeopathic ones like Kamillosan and Calendula cream can be applied after a feed and allowed to soak into the skin. Then there is no need to wash your breasts before the next feed. Creams containing lanolin will need washing off before feeding.

Fresh air will help soreness too. Either sit bra-less for a few minutes after each feed, or if you are very sore you can use two plastic tea strainers (with their handles clipped off) inside your bra between feeds. It sounds funny but it really does work!

DEMAND FEEDING

Most mothers demand feed their babies. This simply means that you feed the baby whenever he wants to be fed. It's the system that nature intended us to use and will help ensure that you have plenty of milk. The more your baby suckles the more milk your body will make. Most babies will take from both breasts at each feed. (A few will only want one breast each time.) Begin on the breast you finished on last time since the baby will suck more enthusiastically from the first breast. Put a safety pin in your bra to remind you which side to start on.

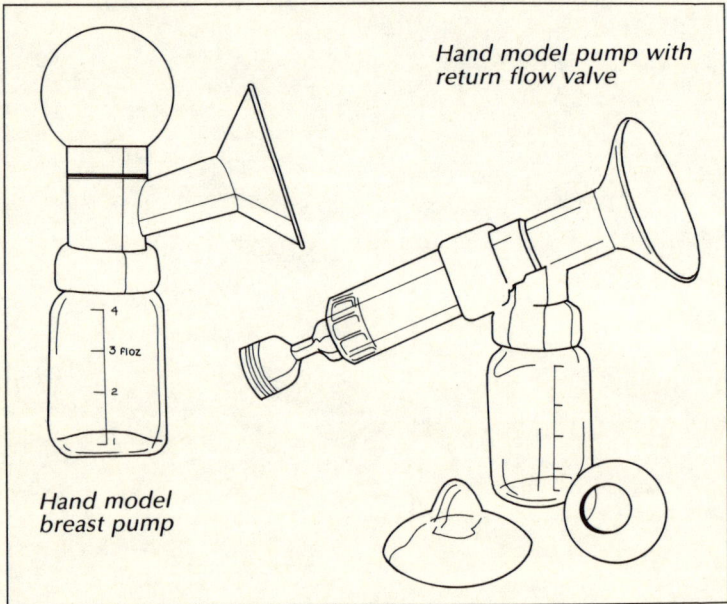

Hand model pump with return flow valve

Hand model breast pump

EXPRESSING MILK

If you have too much milk for comfort or want to leave your baby a supply of milk while you are out or at work you can express some. Hand expressing is a knack that a lot of mothers pick up quickly. You can also try a breast pump. Some of these are rather harsh and can make your nipples sore even when breast feeding is well established. Those with bottles that fit onto the pump make collecting milk easier. Hand pumps with a return flow valve are easier to use if you plan to express milk regularly and they are the gentlest too. Large electric ones are very expensive but can be hired and are useful if your baby is too small or ill to feed directly from your breast. Hospitals have them or they can be hired. Contact your local branch of the National Childbirth Trust; ring 01–221–3833 to find a local breast feeding counsellor.

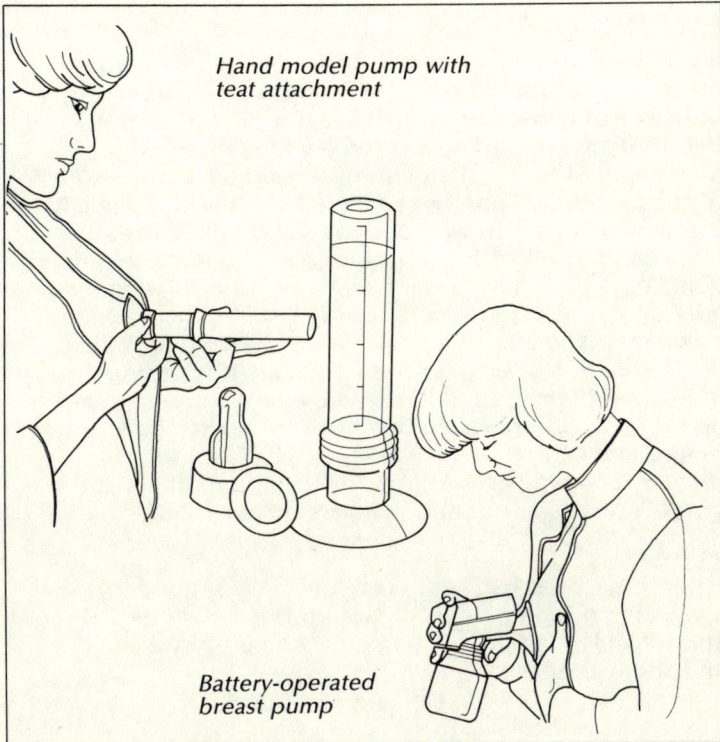

Hand model pump with teat attachment

Battery-operated breast pump

Expressed milk can be stored in a sterilised bottle in the fridge for 24 hours or frozen for three to six months. It's always useful to have some expressed milk in the freezer for the baby if you want to go out for the evening or if you are unwell. If you plan to go back to work you can build up a good stock of milk in the first few weeks when often there is a natural excess of milk. Either store it in plastic bottles or sterilise an ice cube tray, place it inside a plastic bag and seal with a twist tie. Each time you have milk to spare pop it in one of the ice cube sections. When the tray is full tip the 'milk cubes' into a clean plastic bag and seal. Then when you want to leave milk for the baby you can simply 'post' sufficient milk cubes into the bottle and leave it ready for the baby sitter to give. Do a practice run with ordinary ice cubes to make sure that the cubes will fit through the top of the bottle. You may have to make them a little smaller than usual.

FINDING OUT MORE

It's well worth reading more on breast feeding. Two excellent paperback books that you may be able to buy or borrow from your library are *Breast is Best* by Andrew and Penny Stanway and *The Breastfeeding Book* by Marie Messenger. There's plenty of help around for the breast feeding mother. Your midwife and health visitor will advise you and sit with you whilst you feed. The NCT breast feeding counsellors are available to any mother who needs help. You don't have to be a member or have attended NCT classes to ring them. They often will supply and fit nursing bras and keep a stock of aids like nipple shields, homoeopathic creams, and special teats for feeding breast fed babies expressed milk. Local contact numbers can often be found in libraries your local citizens advice bureau or by ringing the central office (01–221–3833). The La Lèche League runs regular meetings for feeding mothers and will give telephone advice too (address on page 153).

TEATS

Often breast fed babies prefer a specially shaped teat that allows them to imitate the action of breast feeding. These are available from many NCT breast feeding counsellors and some chemists.

BOTTLE FEEDING

If you prefer to bottle feed your baby you are likely to need at least six bottles and teats and some method of sterilising them. Only use baby formula milk powder which has been specially adapted to suit a baby. Many new parents find the simplest system is to make up a day's supply of bottles and store them covered in the fridge until needed.

Make up the feeds using cooled boiled water. Rinse each bottle and teat with a little cooled boiled water too. Put the right amount of water in the bottle and then add the measured milk powder. Don't be tempted to add extra powder, or press it down in the scoop as this will alter the composition of the milk. Once the powder is in the bottle, put on the lid and shake well.

When you need a bottle of milk, stand it in a jug of hot water. Keep the teat out of the water and covered with the teat cover. Shake once or twice while it is warming. Check that the milk is not too hot before giving it to the baby, by dripping a little on the inside of your wrist. Throw away any milk left after the feed.

Don't add sugar or rusk to a baby's milk feed: both can make your baby overweight. Babies may also need cooled boiled water to drink especially in hot weather.

If you go out for the day, carry the milk ready-prepared in the bottle, but keep it cool. If necessary carry a flask of hot water to use for warming it up. Never be tempted to keep the milk warm as bacteria can grow very rapidly in warm milk. Most restaurants and cafés are quite happy to supply hot water for warming bottles.

It's tempting to use a microwave oven for warming bottles of milk. However, the heating pattern is often uneven, with hot and cold spots developing. If you do use a microwave oven to heat the milk shake it well and leave it for a couple of minutes to allow the temperature to equalise.

STERILISING KITS

For bottle feeding, a chemical sterilising kit is useful. This is a large plastic tank that holds the bottles, teats, collars and bottle covers. The sterilising solution comes as a liquid, tablet or granular form. It needs to be made up freshly each day and the bottles etc. take about 30 minutes to be sterilised. Bottles can be stored in the solution until needed and plastic beaker cups, plates and spoons can also be sterilised in it. Metal utensils should not be placed in chemical sterilisers.

It's important to wash and rinse the bottles well before putting them in the sterilising solution. Teats should be cleaned inside with a little salt which will loosen the milk scum. Rinse well to remove all traces of salt. Also make sure they are fully immersed. Most sterilising kits have a plate to hold the bottles down under the water level.

Rinse bottles and teats with cooled boiled water after sterilising them in chemical solutions.

Some parents develop an allergy to the solution so a pair of plastic tongs may be useful to avoid contact with the liquid.

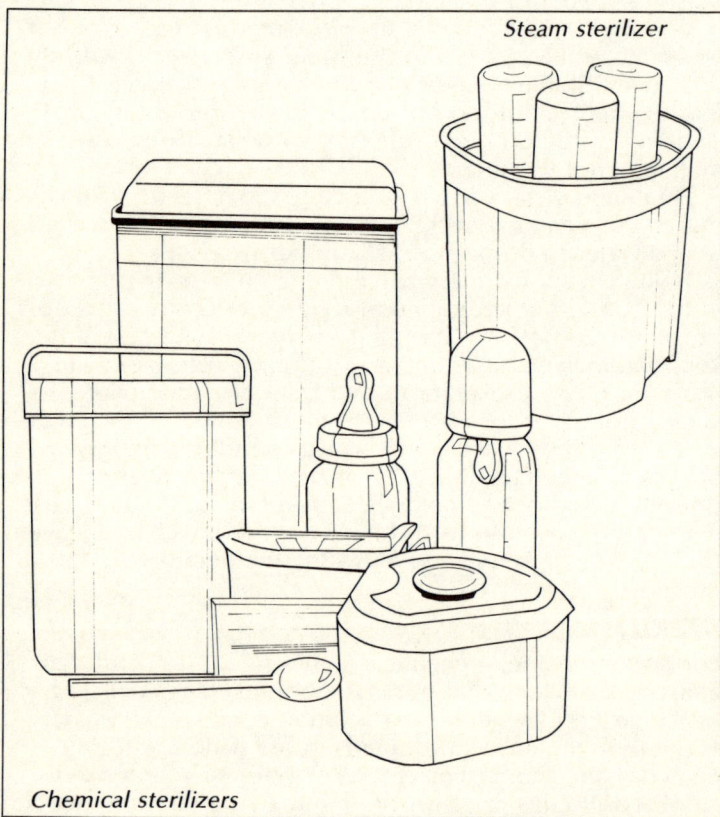

Steam sterilizer

Chemical sterilizers

Steam sterilisers are expensive at the moment as they are quite new. They are however, very fast and will sterilise teats and bottles in five minutes. They are compact electric devices that plug in and can stand on a worktop. They are useful to anyone allergic to the sterilising solution or anyone who wants to get bottles ready quickly.

If you only occasionally need to sterilise bottles, consider buying a smaller than average sterilising kit or using a plastic ice-cream tub. This will take one or two bottles plus teats and collars. Measure the water carefully and use the right amount of sterilising granules or liquid to get the correct strength. You will need to hold the bottles under the water and allow the air to bubble out to make sure there are no air bubbles inside.

Boiling is another method of sterilising. Keep an old pan specially for this and boil everything for ten minutes, then allow to cool before handling them.

Again it's tempting to use the microwave to sterilise bottles, but because of the cold spot problem it is not advisable. In one set of tests it was shown that bottles sterilised in a microwave oven had several unsterile spots in them.

BOTTLES AND TEATS

Wide-necked plastic bottles are the most commonly used nowadays. These are easy to fill and won't break if dropped. Most hold around 250 ml (8 to 9 fl oz) but smaller ones are available (125 ml/4 fl oz). These are useful for giving cooled boiled water or diluted fruit juice once the baby is a few weeks old.

Most bottles have a screw collar to hold the teat on and a teat cover to keep it clean. An inner plastic disc that fits under the teat seals the bottle and prevents spillages. Some bottles are wide enough to take a screw-on beaker lid for use as your baby becomes old enough to cope with drinking from a spout.

Bottles with disposable liners are available too. These are designed to minimise the air the baby takes in, as the polythene liner collapses as the baby drinks the milk. They are useful for colicky babies and for babies who are usually breast fed.

Teats are available in various shapes and sizes. Some teats are shaped to resemble a mother's breast to make sucking from a teat easier for a baby who is usually breast fed.

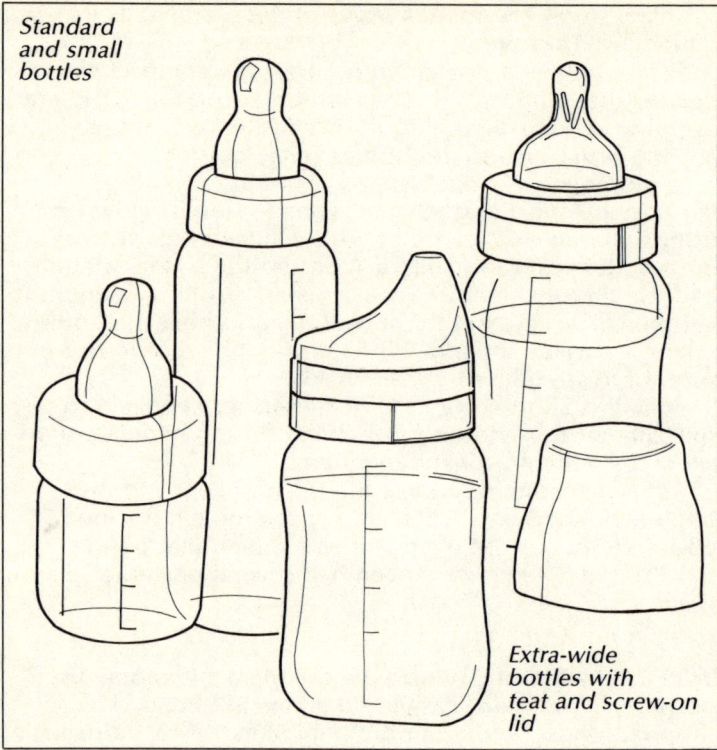

Standard and small bottles

Extra-wide bottles with teat and screw-on lid

Teats are usually sold with small, medium and large holes. As your baby grows and sucks more energetically you may find you need to change the hole size.

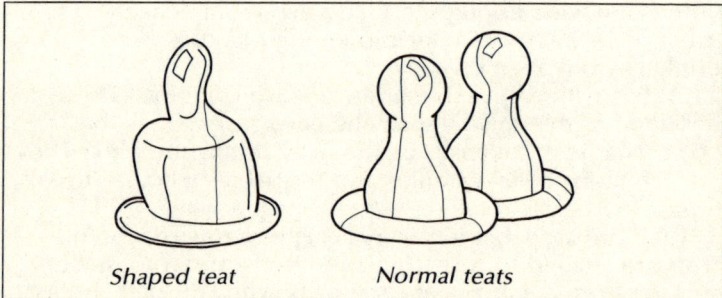

Shaped teat   Normal teats

INTRODUCING SOLIDS

At around four to six months, most babies are ready to begin trying small amounts of solid foods. This stage is entirely different from 'weaning' which comes much later. For some months your baby will still need milk feeds as well as solid foods. As he eats more solids so he will gradually drop the milk feeds.

Some foods should be avoided at first particularly those high in salt, and those likely to cause allergies.

FOODS TO AVOID WHEN FIRST INTRODUCING SOLIDS

FOOD	PROBLEM	WHEN TO INTRODUCE
Egg White	Common cause of allergies.	Eight months at the earliest.
Pipped soft fruits e.g. strawberries, raspberries	Common cause of allergies.	Eight months at the earliest.
Cow's Milk	Can cause allergies for some children. Delay introduction and then boil and dilute with cooled boiled water if there is a family history of allergy or eczema or asthma.	Six months at earliest, twelve months preferably.
Sugar and sweetened syrups	Sugar is fattening and bad for the teeth. Avoid adding it to baby foods as it will encourage a sweet tooth to develop.	Avoid as long as possible. Use naturally sweet foods such as dried fruits, to add sweetness. Opt for unrefined sugars for baking.

FOOD	PROBLEM	WHEN TO INTRODUCE
Bacon/ham and similar products	All high in nitrates.	Wait as long as possible: until 18 months to two years.
Salt and salted foods	Too much salt in the diet is bad for children and adults.	Avoid as long as possible.
Spinach	Naturally high in nitrates. These are usually eliminated through the kidneys and small babies have immature kidneys.	Wait as long as possible: until 18 months to two years.
Pro-cessed and refined foods	These often have additives in them. Some additives are banned from baby foods but allowed in foods intended for adults.	Avoid as long as possible.
Honey	Rare form of botulism (food poisoning) has been caused by honey in some countries.	Avoid for the first year.
Wheat based foods e.g. rusks, cereal based foods, oats, bread	Some babies are sensitive to gluten in wheat (coeliac dis-ease). It is thought that early introduction of gluten may trigger this off. Look for the gluten-free symbol.	Avoid until six months.

FIRST FOODS: FOUR TO SIX MONTHS

At first babies need just little tastes of food. Offer them after the milk feed at lunchtime or teatime. If your baby is not interested, wait a few days and then try again. It's worth introducing just one food at a time. Then if your baby shows any adverse reaction you will know which food is the likely cause. Try an eating apple, cooked in a little water then puréed, or vegetables such as carrot or cauliflower. Thin the purée with extra cooled boiled water, with formula milk or expressed breast milk. Baby rice makes a good bland food and is gluten free.

Many parents find it easier to use prepared baby foods at this stage. It is a lot of effort to produce a tablespoon or so of baby food that your offspring may just spit back at you! If you do choose to use packet foods or jars or tins, read the labels carefully. Some have added sugar, or dried skimmed milk added to them. There are many available that do not. Jars of pure fruit, simply cooked and puréed, are ideal first foods. Many packets have detailed labelling on the front highlighting such points as 'no sugar', 'gluten free', 'lactose free' or 'suitable for vegetarians'.

TEXTURE

The texture of the food is very important. It needs to be very smooth and quite thin. After all your baby has only experienced milk before, so he will have to learn to cope with this new substance. Most foods need to be liquidised and then sieved. Later just liquidising will suffice.

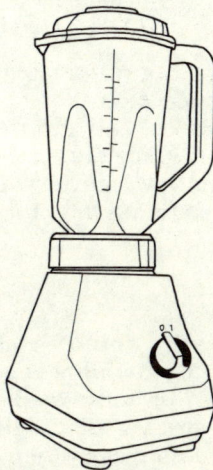

Liquidizer

A liquidiser or food processor is useful here, or opt for a hand-held blender, a non-electric food mouli or simply a sieve and wooden spoon. A special baby blender is available with jars for storing the food in.

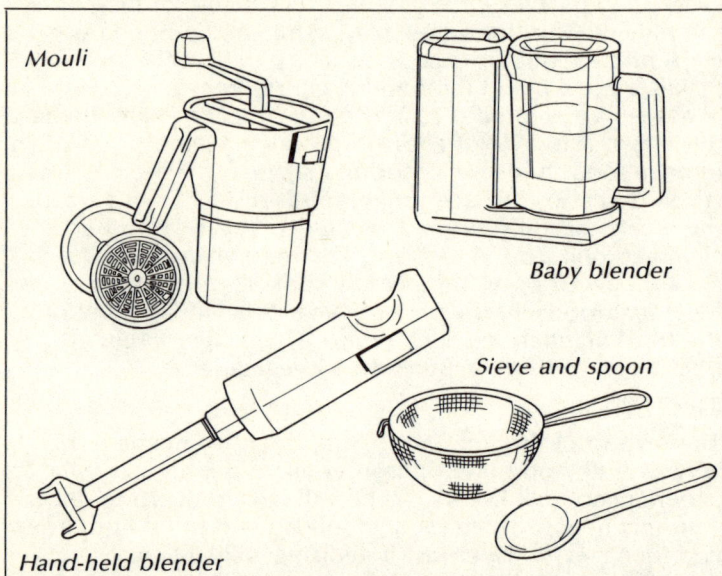

Mouli

Baby blender

Sieve and spoon

Hand-held blender

THE NEXT STEP: SIX TO EIGHT MONTHS

Once your baby is taking reasonable amounts of food it becomes more practical to make everything yourself. Special dishes can be cooked and frozen ready for use. Purées can be frozen in ice cube trays, so that you can thaw just enough food whenever you need it. Or save yoghurt pots and margarine tubs for freezing larger amounts.

RECIPE IDEAS

Vegetable Casserole

Peel and chop a selection of fresh vegetables, such as potato, carrot, parsnip, cauliflower and a little leek or onion. Cook in water or home-made stock until very tender. Do not use stock cubes as these are usually very salty and may have additives in them. Purée. Freeze in small tubs.

Cheesey Lentils
Cook 200 g/8 oz of dried red lentils in 200 ml/$\frac{3}{4}$ pt of water.
Simmer until most of the water is absorbed and the lentils
are very soft. Beat well with a wooden spoon to make a soft
purée. Freeze in individual portions. Once thawed and
reheated, sprinkle a little finely grated cheese on top.

Recipe Books
It's worth buying or borrowing a good recipe book for baby
foods. Two I would recommend are *Growing Up With
Good Food* by Catherine Lewis (Unwin Paperbacks) and
The Right Food For Your Kids by Lousie Templeton
(Century) which is particularly good for vegetarian recipes.
As your baby grows my book *Healthy Cooking for Children*
(Marks and Spencer) includes good family food with
instructions for modifying recipes for children.

EIGHT MONTHS ONWARDS

By this stage many babies are keen to feed themselves and
can cope with finger foods: try rusks, thin fingers of fruits
such as pear, apple or banana or vegetables such as carrot
and cucumber. Finely grated cheese, carrot or apple is ideal
for babies who can't quite cope with fingers of food.
Grated in a mouli grater, the texture and shape are ideal for
small babies. In our house cheese grated in this way is
called 'round and round' cheese since the grater handle
goes round and round to produce it!

To encourage your baby to feed himself, shaped bowls
and cutlery are available. Bowls that stick to the high chair

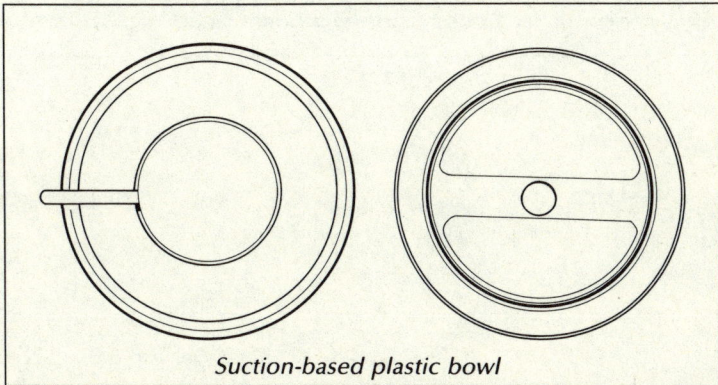

Suction-based plastic bowl

tray and have shaped sides to allow the baby to push the food onto the spoon are a good idea. Cutlery shaped to allow the baby to grip it, and turned slightly inwards to make aiming for his mouth easier are also a good buy. Start with two spoons and then progress to a spoon and a fork.

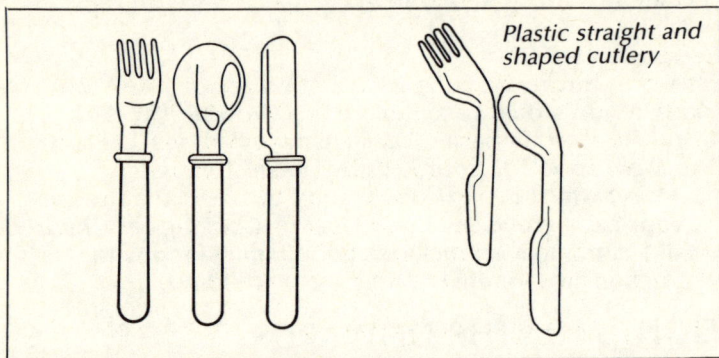

Plastic straight and shaped cutlery

Plastic cutlery is better than metal at first. It's less likely to hurt emerging teeth and sore gums, and it can be popped into sterilising solution to clean it.

By this stage, bibs with arms are a good idea.

DRINKS

Avoid syrups containing sugar. Instead use pure fruit juices well diluted with cooled boiled water. Special baby juices using a combination of fruits for natural sweetness are also available. Water alone can be used and some babies like herbal drinks like fennel. These can be offered in a bottle, on a spoon or in a cup. Choose a beaker cup with a narrow

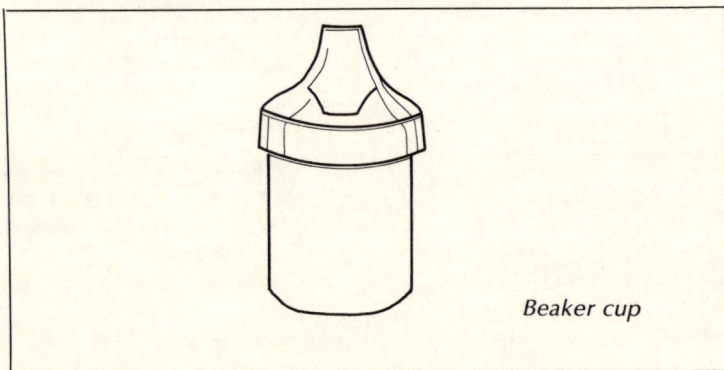

Beaker cup

spout and fine holes as a first cup. Large holes can allow the liquid out too quickly for the baby to cope with at first.

TEETHING

It is tempting to blame every crying bout, nappy rash, red cheek and raised temperature on teething. Many babies cut their teeth with little or no trouble. Others are fretful and grumpy, with sore gums accompanied by copious dribbling. It is always worth checking with your health visitor or doctor if your baby is off colour, even if he is teething. It may well be that he has an ear infection or other ailment at the same time. So eliminate other possible causes of distress first and then turn your attention to making him as comfortable as possible.

Many babies do like to bite and chew on the gum as their teeth are coming through. Rusks sometimes help, although many contain rather a lot of sugar. Teething rings can be useful too. Choose ones that are soft with some give in them. Some are very hard and hurt tender gums. Rings that can be chilled can give some comfort. Only ever chill them in the 'fridge, not the freezer. If they are too cold they could burn a baby's skin or gums.

Teething gels sometimes help. Often, though, it is the sensation of having the gums rubbed that helps as much as anything else. Homoeopathic teething granules are useful too. They can be used quite frequently with no fear of side-effects, and many babies like them.

If your baby is really in pain, a pain killer at night may help everyone to sleep. Check with your doctor first to eliminate other causes. Many parents worry about giving a pain killer, but it can be very helpful on a short-term basis. Always use one suitable for babies, and do **not** give aspirin or aspirin-based products; your health visitor will advise which brand to use. Some teething gels should not be used in conjunction with a pain killer so check on the tube.

BATHING

Bathing a new born baby can be quite worrying — they seem so tiny and wriggly. All new parents think they are going to drop their baby. It is really another of those parenting skills that you pick up very quickly. Usually newborns are bathed every day, so it's worth getting organised. You can buy a baby bath and stand, or a folding changing table with a bath fitted to it. Baths that fit over the main bath are useful as you don't have to carry water around. However, there are other cheaper alternatives. Try using a washing up bowl. Spread towels on the floor in front of the fire and place the bowl on the floor. Then you can lay out all the things you need and kneel down to wash the baby. Or use the kitchen sink. It is just about the right size and height. Once washed the baby can be lifted onto towels on the draining board. Wrap an old towel around the taps to prevent them dripping or the baby touching them.

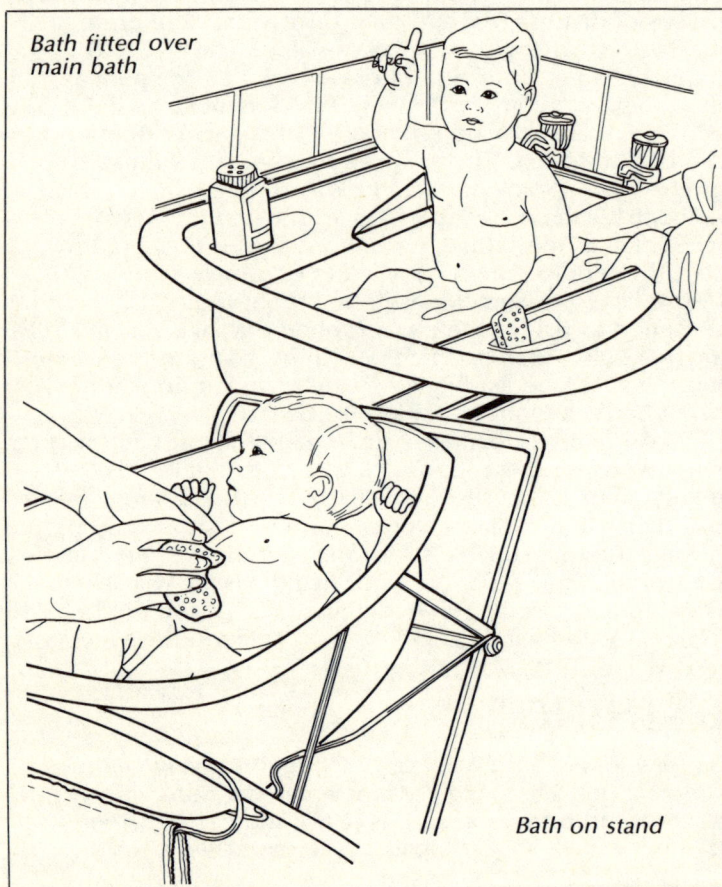

Bath fitted over main bath

Bath on stand

Liquid soap (which is added to the bath water) avoids having to hold onto a bar of soap and the baby.

Supports for bathing new born babies are available. These are either shaped foam wedges or a towelling-covered frame which hold the baby at an angle. Some baths have shaped bases to support the baby as well.

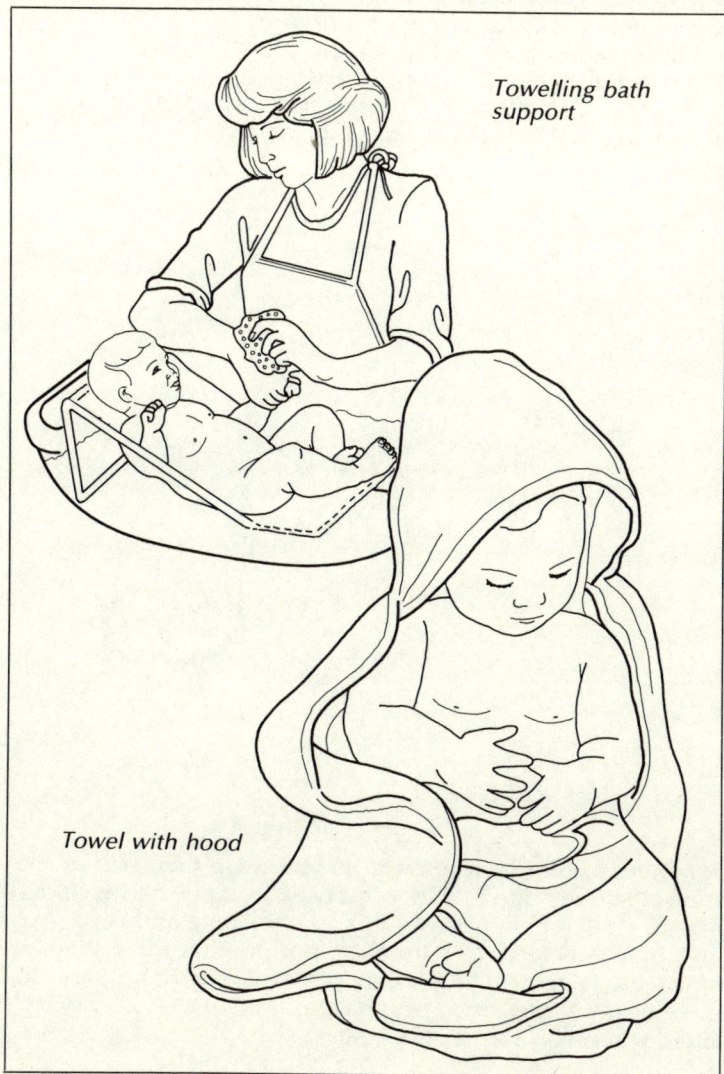

Towelling bath support

Towel with hood

HAIR WASHING

With a tiny baby hair washing is reasonably simple. Wrap the baby in a warm bath towel so that he cannot wriggle too much, and then lay him across your lap with his head over the bath. Wet and wash his hair, then rinse and rub dry. Babies lose a lot of heat through their heads, so don't leave his hair wet for any length of time.

Older babies that are too big or wriggly to hold are more of a handful. Often propping a plastic baby mirror at the end of the bath helps. You can shampoo his hair and let him watch as you make horns with the soapy hair.

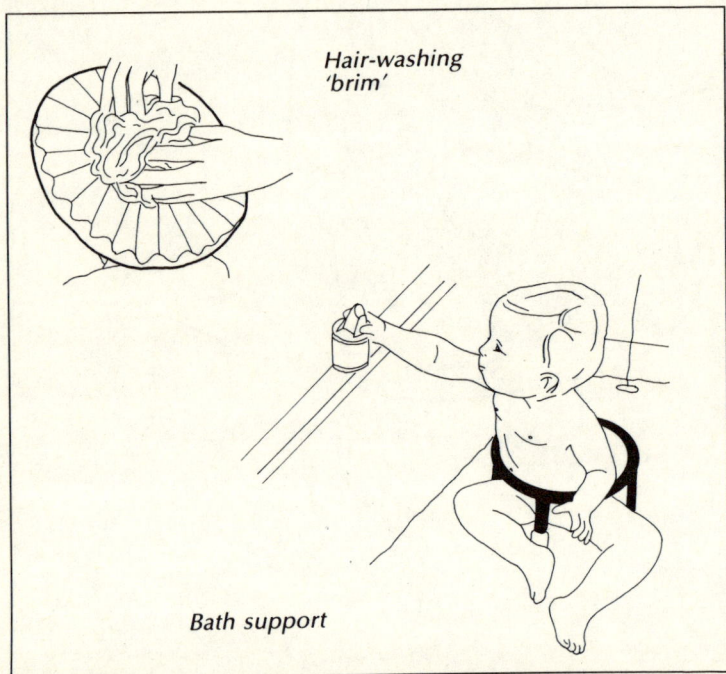

Hair-washing
'brim'

Bath support

Sometimes older children will let you wash their hair in the shower as they don't have to lie back in the water to have it rinsed. If your child really hates hair washing and it's a screaming session every time, try not doing it for a couple of weeks. They won't look very pretty, but it won't harm to leave it unwashed, and they may just forget that they were afraid when you start again.

PRACTICAL TIPS FOR BATH TIME

1. Always have everything ready. Line up towels, cotton wool, nappy, cream, pins, clothes etc. beside the bath and double check so you don't forget anything vital.

2. Liquid soap (added to the water) is easier to cope with than the traditional bar of soap, and the baby may prefer it to feeling insecure and slippery when soaped.

3. Check the temperature of the water very carefully. Adult hands are not very sensitive so use your elbow or the soft skin on the inside of your arm instead.

4. Baby baths full of water weigh a great deal. Either stand the baby bath inside the main bath, or fill it with a jug. This is very important during the first few weeks after having a baby, and particularly so if you have had a Caesarian section.

5. If your baby's skin is very dry, try adding a little oil to the bath instead of soap. Almond oil is ideal. Ask at your chemists for the unbranded type which is very cheap.

6. Never be tempted to leave your child in the bath, even for a few seconds. Ignore the 'phone or doorbell, or take your baby out of the water and wrap him in a towel.

7. Have a spare towel on your lap before picking the baby up, or use a towelling apron with a plastic backing. Even if he is wrapped in a towel the dampness soaks through.

8. Use talcum powder sparingly if at all. Excessive amounts can make your baby cough and splutter, and it can cake in the creases of his body.

9. Dry your baby carefully. Babies have lots of creases where the water collects and these need careful drying.

10. Some babies hate being bathed. They don't have to be given daily baths. 'Top and tail' instead — washing the baby's head, neck and chest with cotton wool balls, then drying and dressing him, before washing his bottom and legs. Or try taking him in the bath with you. Often the skin to skin contact gives him confidence. Make sure the water is the right temperature for him though.

CRYING

All babies cry at some time: it's their only form of communication. Sometimes the cry means, 'I'm hungry or thirsty', sometimes it means, 'I'm uncomfortable', and sometimes it's a lonely cry from a baby that's bored or needs a cuddle. Many babies cry because they are tired and need to settle down in their cot or crib. The secret is knowing just what each cry means! It often takes weeks before you understand your baby's cries, and there are undoubtedly days when nothing you can do soothes him.

Generally it is worth working through the possibilities and dealing with practical points first like is he hungry, thirsty, wet or dirty? Wind can plague some babies. Often you can feel it rumbling around in their tummies or see them drawing their legs up and down in pain. Homoeopathic teething granules or a fennel drink may help; gripe water rarely does. Some babies are prone to colic. This tends to set in at a certain time each day and your usually happy baby begins to cry heartily for long periods. It is usually outgrown by three to four months, but in the meantime life can be fraught. Some breast-feeding mothers find it helps to eliminate dairy products and eggs from their diet. A dummy sometimes helps too, as a baby with colic generally wants to suck all the time and this can create a vicious circle: the more he feeds, the more his tummy hurts. Consult your health visitor and doctor as they may be able to suggest suitable medication too.

COMFORTING AND CRYING

There seem to be three elements that can help comfort a crying baby: movement, sound and touch. Rocking a baby up and down often soothes him. A rocking chair is a comfortable way of doing this. Or try pushing him in the pram, or an automatic crib rocker which bounces the crib in a net suspended from a hook. Walking up and down soothes some babies, or sit them on your hip and gently sway back and forth.

Sounds can soothe too. Tapes of 'womb noises' or 'white noise' are available. They need to be started within the first ten weeks to be effective. Some parents find that the noise of the vacuum cleaner or washing machine will distract or soothe a baby too. Singing to your baby often helps and is usually much more pleasant to listen to than machine noises! Sometimes a father's deep voice and the vibration the baby can feel when held against his chest and neck work wonders.

Touch is very important to babies and adults alike. A 'baby sheepskin' will help some babies to settle and can be

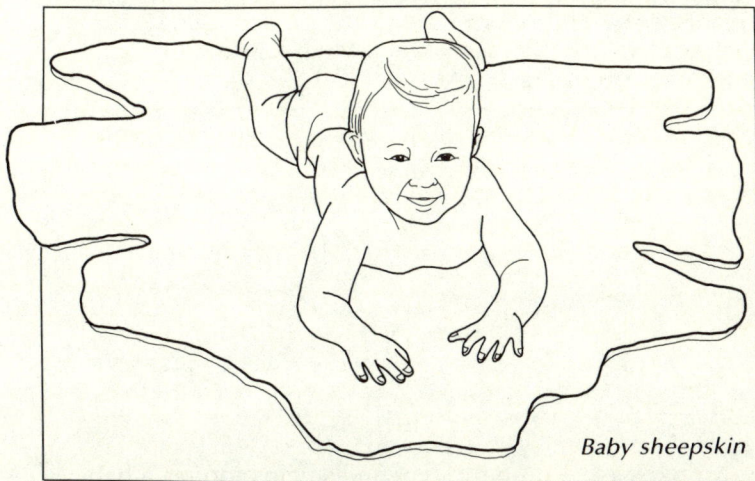

Baby sheepskin

used in a crib, cot or pram. Later it can also be used on the floor, for the baby to be on while playing. Skin to skin contact helps too, and many fathers find their offspring dropping off to sleep while lying on dad's chest. In fact, fathers can often comfort a breast-fed baby when the mother cannot. This is simply because the baby can smell the mother's milk, and while he may not be hungry the smell attracts him and makes him want to suck.

Carrying or holding the baby in certain ways sometimes seems to help too. Nervous, fractious babies seem to like being tightly swaddled, others dislike having their arms too tightly bound. Some like being carried around in a sling. Windy babies may feel better up on your shoulder or laid over your knees while you rock them gently to and fro. Many like a steady regular pat on the back. Experiment to see what suits your baby best.

If your baby is tired, it may just be that he needs a few minutes in his cot to wind down and drop off to sleep. Try putting him to bed and then going downstairs for a cup of coffee before going back to him. It sometimes does the trick and makes you less tense when you go back.

Babies that cry constantly may well have an allergy or be ill in some way, so do take advice from your health visitor or doctor. Support for a new parent with a crying baby is vital. It's all too easy to feel inadequate, frustrated and alone. Other local parents can help. Try the following organisations who offer local mutual support: Crysis, National Childbirth Trust, Meet-a-Mum Association (addresses on pages 153–4).

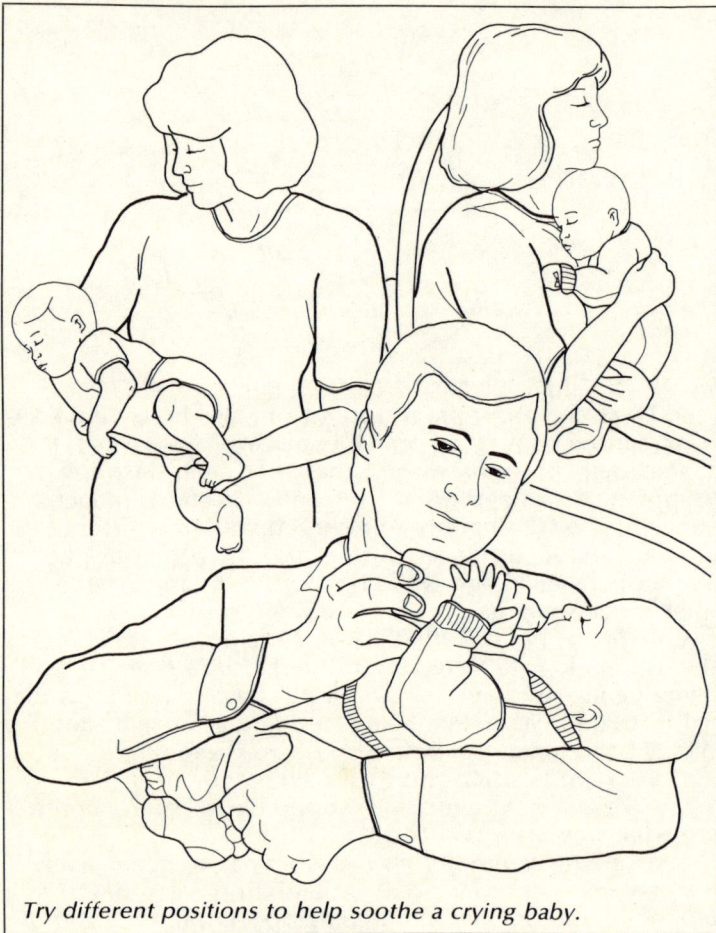

Try different positions to help soothe a crying baby.

TIPS ON COPING WITH A CRYING BABY

1. Always make sure that the baby is physically comfortable before you try anything else. He may be hungry or thirsty; wet or dirty; too hot or too cold; in a draught; the bedding may be damp or crumpled.
2. Wind can be a problem. To ease wind, hold the baby on your shoulder and rub his back gently but firmly.
3. Colic is more difficult to ease; if it is serious, you should consult your health visitor or doctor. In the meantime, try wrapping a warm hot water bottle in a towel, placing it on your knees and laying the baby comfortably on top. You can also use warmed towels. Try a fennel drink.
4. Try music, noise or talking.
5. Rocking, walking or pushing in the pram sometimes helps.
6. Fresh air can calm a crying baby, as long as it is not too cold. It also does wonders for your own nerves.
7. Take turns with your husband to try to comfort the baby. Try to get out of earshot and relax with a warm drink, a hot bath or perhaps a small sherry!
8. Take the baby for a drive in the car.
9. Give the baby a warm bath.
10. Some babies just like to be cuddled. Try to find a comfortable position where you are both relaxed. The baby may also like to be gently stroked, and this is also soothing for the parents. Skin to skin contact can work, or a baby sheepskin.
11. Try a dummy.
12. Put the baby in a sling.

CLOTHES AND SHOES

Dressing your baby can be great fun, especially while they are too young to have any say over what they wear. Once they are old enough to choose you spend all your life trying to persuade your two-year-old that shorts and a T-shirt are not the best thing to wear on a chilly December morning! So enjoy this earlier stage of being able to choose for them.

Baby clothes need to be warm, comfortable, and easy to get on and off. Once they are crawling they also need to be robust enough to withstand the hard wear they will receive. In general, natural fabrics are best, and a fabric with a slight stretch is more comfortable and easier to get on and off. Poppers are easier than buttons, and ties and ribbons are a nuisance.

The traditional layette, all hand-made during pregnancy in readiness for the baby's arrival, has largely disappeared now. That's partly because we now dress boys and girls slightly differently even from birth. In days gone past boys were dressed in exactly the same frilly dresses and suits as girls, so a layette would suit either sex.

VESTS AND STRETCH SUITS

It's well worth having several vests and stretch baby suits before the baby arrives. Then with gifts of knitted cardigans, hats and mittens etc. you will be able to cope for the first few days and buy extras as needed.

Envelope opening vests are much simpler than tie vests, which always manage to come undone. Long-sleeved vests seem a good idea. However, as soon as you try to put something on over the top the sleeve tangles up. It is then hard to sort it out and make it comfortable for the baby. Vests with poppers that do up under the nappy are easy to put on, and help keep the nappy in place. They stop any waist-level draughts as well. They are available in towelling or cotton and can be machine washed — another prerequisite for baby clothes. Buy four to six of them.

Stretch suits of the all-in-one kind keep the baby warm and comfortable without restricting his movements. These are available in plain white or in pretty colours and patterns. Again they wash well and don't need ironing. Buy half a dozen of these. Some have turnback mittens on the arms to keep the baby's hands warm or to stop him scratching himself. Make sure that there is plenty of room for the baby's feet. Tight stretch suits can damage developing feet.

Babies do lose quite a lot of heat through their heads, so hats are useful, especially if your's is a winter baby. Mittens and bootees help keep extremities warm too. Make sure that any knitted mittens are quite closely knitted or your baby's fingers can slip through the knitted holes.

Stretch suits make ideal sleeping suits. Some parents like to use nighties too. Look for nighties with a drawstring at the bottom hem. These keep the baby warm and prevent

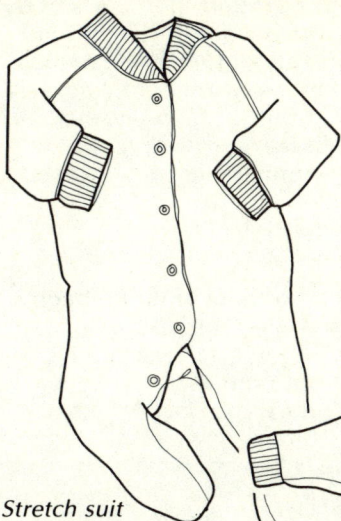

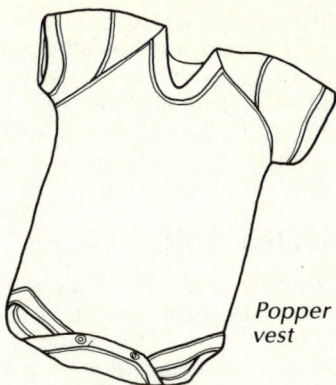

Popper vest

Stretch suit

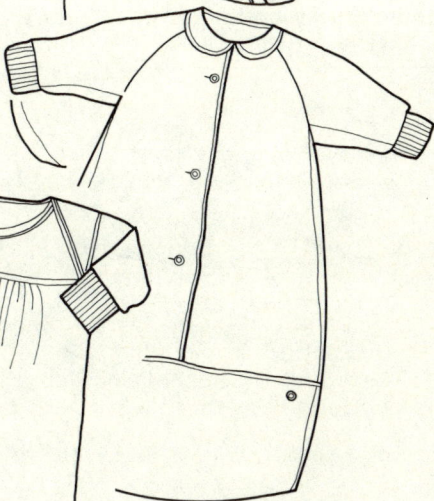

Sleeping bag

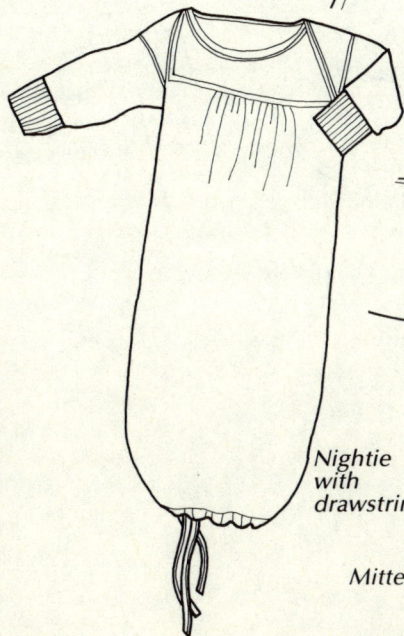

Nightie with drawstring

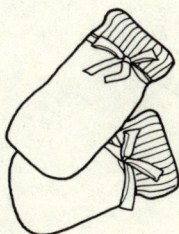

Mittens

the nightie lifting up and tangling around the baby's body. Sleeping bags, with a hooded top and set-in sleeves, are useful if you want to take your baby out in the evenings, or for walks on very cold days. They are worn over a stretch suit or nightie and keep him warm even if you want to lift him out of his pram or Moses basket for feeding. Some babies find these too warm for normal night-time sleeps in a centrally-heated house, however.

SHOES AND SOCKS

It's not worth buying shoes for your baby until he begins to walk. Before then bootees or towelling slippers will keep his feet warm. Slipper socks are useful for crawling babies. These have a plastic sole sewn onto the sock and they generally stay on longer than ordinary socks.

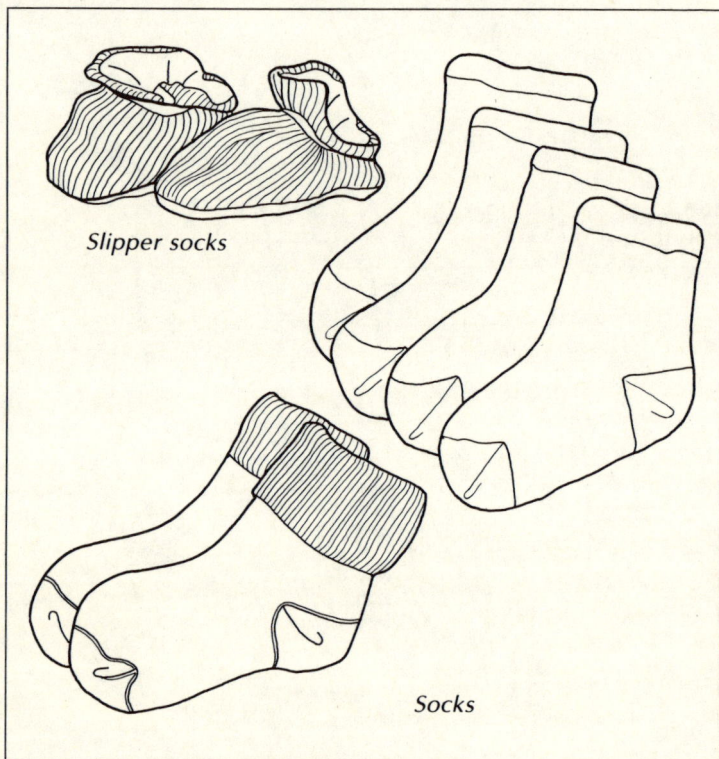

Slipper socks

Socks

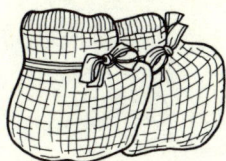

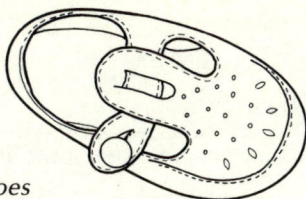

Shoes

Real shoes need careful measuring. Go to a shoe shop which has specially trained assistants. Even in winter it's worth choosing a really lightweight shoe at first as your baby is likely to find his first shoes feel very heavy. Ensure his socks fit well too. The bones in the feet are very soft and easily damaged by socks and shoes that are too small. Have his feet re-measured every three months or so. Buy cheap, well-fitting shoes frequently rather than expensive shoes infrequently.

COATS

An all-in-one oversuit is a more practical buy than a winter coat for a tiny baby. It will keep him warm and still allow him to move around. They are available in lightweight waterproof materials or with warm linings for winter wear.

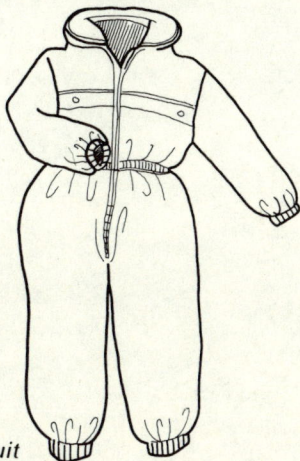

All-in-one oversuit

For tiny babies choose one with built-in feet. For older children look for one with elasticated cuffs around the ankles and sleeves.

All-in-one oversuits with feet for smaller babies and without for toddlers

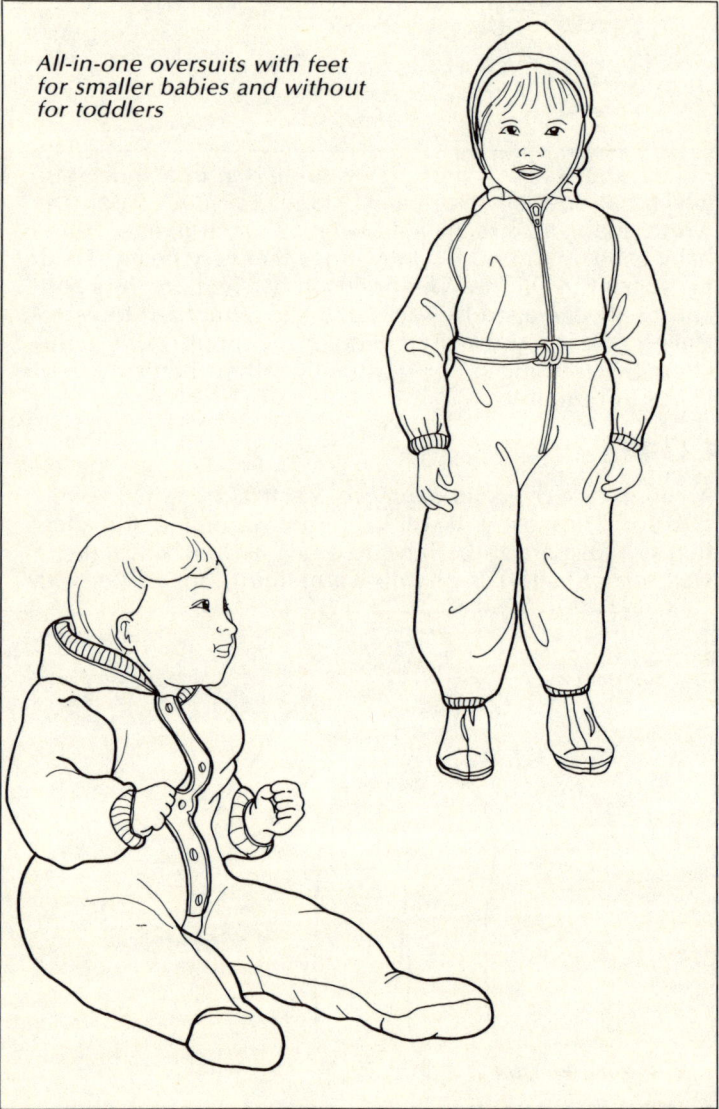

CLOTHES FOR CRAWLING AND PLAYING

At this stage it is vital to choose practical clothes. Dresses will restrict a little girl and may trip her up, so keep them for high days and holidays. Dungarees are the best bet, as trousers tend to slip down and shirts then untuck. Buy two or three pairs of tough dungarees in slightly stretchy fabric, so that as your baby tries to crawl or reach up for things the clothes give slightly. Crawling clothes usually get very dirty and wear out on the knees. It may be worth adding extra patches to the knees before they are worn. Then as the patches wear out you can replace them. It is much easier to sew a new patch on when the material underneath is not worn through.

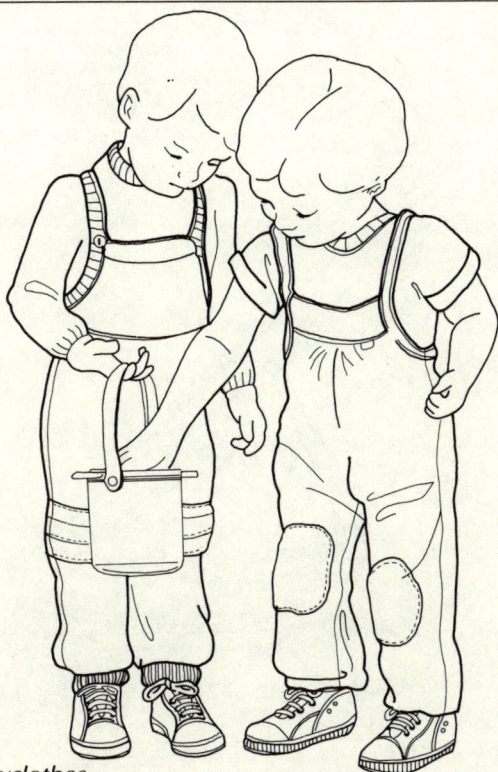

Ideal playclothes

Buggy facing mother

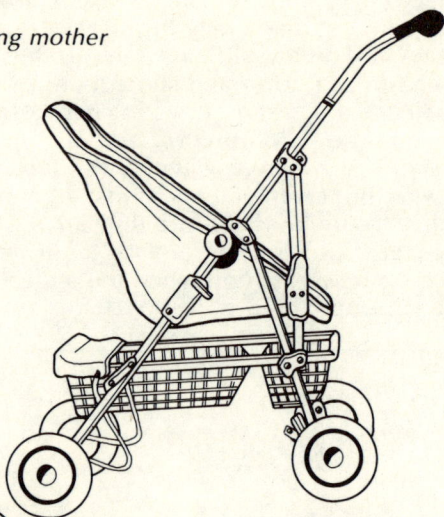

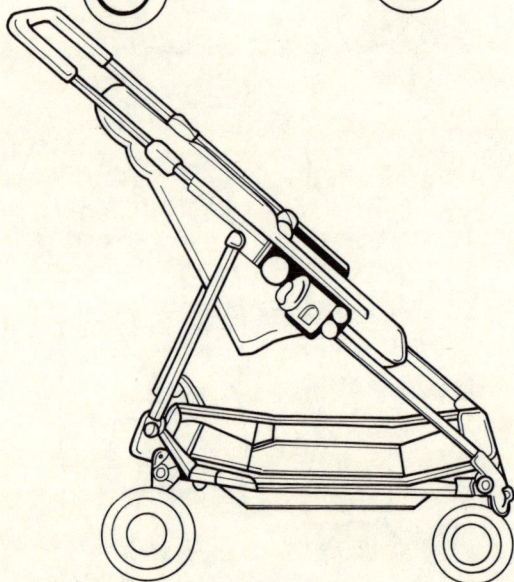

Flat-fold buggy

3 GETTING OUT AND ABOUT

In years gone by most babies were simply carried in their mother's arms, or wrapped around with a shawl until they were big enough to walk. Only the very rich had any form of baby carriages. The first prams were made by carriage builders and the first pushchairs were in fact adapted mail carts. It became the status symbol for late Victorian mothers and their nannies. In the first decade or two of this century folding wooden pushchairs were available for hire at most seaside railway stations for a penny a day.

PRAMS AND PUSHCHAIRS

Now the choice of methods of getting out and about with your baby is very wide. So wide in fact that deciding which type of pram or pushchair, let alone which brand, to choose can be difficult.

Consider your lifestyle. If you live in the country and will have to walk long distances to the shops you are likely to find a large robust pram very useful. Anyone who lives in a flat or needs to hop on and off buses will prefer a lightweight pushchair. Remember that swivel wheels are really designed for paved areas and are not ideal for rough paths or roads.

Carriage-built prams are still popular if somewhat expensive. Smaller versions are now available. Some prams have a flat-based body, usually with a fabric finish. This can double up as a robust carrycot to use in the car whilst the wheels fold for storage. This type of carrycot is usually pretty heavy and not really designed for carrying around much. A carrycot and transporter is lighter and generally folds much smaller. Of course many families choose a fully reclining pushchair which will take a new born baby. Each of these has advantages and disadvantages. Here is a summary of the main points to consider for each.

Soft-bodied pram

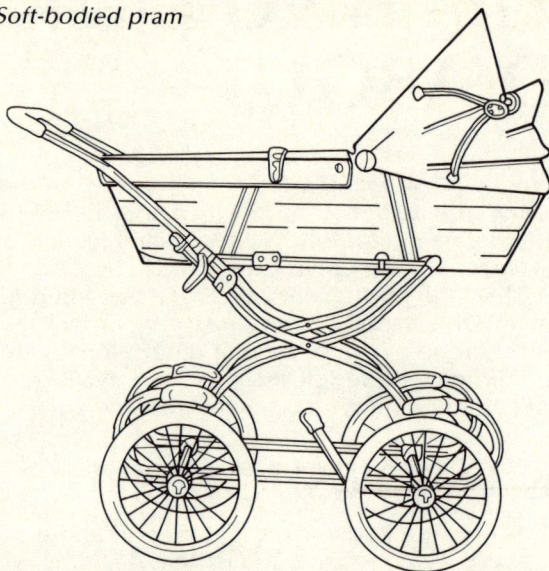

Carrycot and transporter

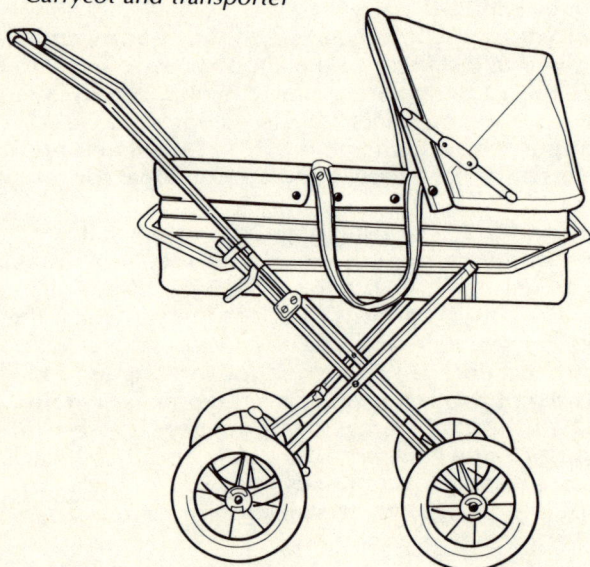

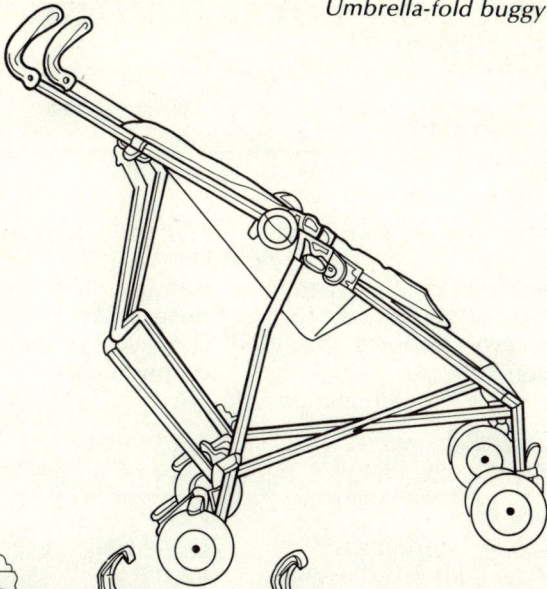

Umbrella-fold buggy

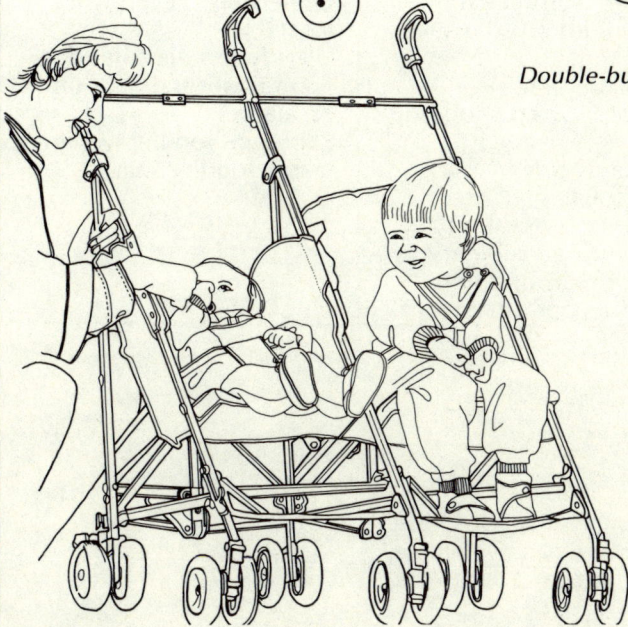

Double-buggy

ADVANTAGES AND DISADVANTAGES OF PRAMS, CARRYCOT TRANSPORTERS AND PUSHCHAIRS

LARGE PRAM	
Pros Easy to push. Comfortable and warm for the baby. Often lasts until the baby is about eighteen months. Can carry shopping underneath. Can use a toddler seat on top.	*Cons* Needs to be stored. Large to get in and out of shops. Cannot fold to go on buses/trains or in cars. Expensive (but available secondhand).
SOFT BODIED PRAM	
Pros Versatile as usually the body will lift off to use as a carrycot. Usually has a reasonable-sized shopping tray. Reasonably priced and wide choice. Usually last until the baby is ready for an ordinary pushchair, around nine months to one year.	*Cons* Quite bulky, even when folded. Usually too big to fold to go in buses/trains or on escalators. Some are too lightweight to take a toddler seat.

CARRYCOT/TRANSPORTER	
Pros Lightweight and usually easy to fold and store. Carrycot will fit in the back of car and can be secured with safety straps. Not too expensive.	*Cons* Not ideal for rough ground or if you will have to walk long distances. Soon outgrown, usually by around six months.
PUSHCHAIRS	
Pros Lightweight. Some can recline to take a new born baby. Easy to fold and carry. Can fit into car/onto bus. Easy to get into shops/lifts.	*Cons* Not very warm for newborns — you need to wrap them up very well. Check that they can be folded with the hood and apron on; some cannot which means dismantling while holding the baby and the shopping. Some have nowhere for shopping; hanging bags on the back of buggies is very dangerous.

Within each range there is considerable variation in the features offered. Look around the shops and ask other mothers what they think about the pushchairs and prams they have. Don't be rushed into a decision. Sleep on it and go back when you have decided.

SAFETY NOTE

Always use a harness to hold the baby in a pram or pushchair. Even when too small to wriggle and climb there is the possibility that the pram might tip over as you go up and down pavements, or an older child may try to climb onto it.

The British Standard on pushchairs now requires them to have linked brakes. This is to prevent one brake coming off and the pushchair swivelling sideways on a hill.

BABIES IN CARS

It is vital to fit and use a proper safety restraint for your baby from the very beginning. Unrestrained babies can be projected out of the car even in quite low-speed crashes. For new born babies the choice is a carrycot or baby seat.

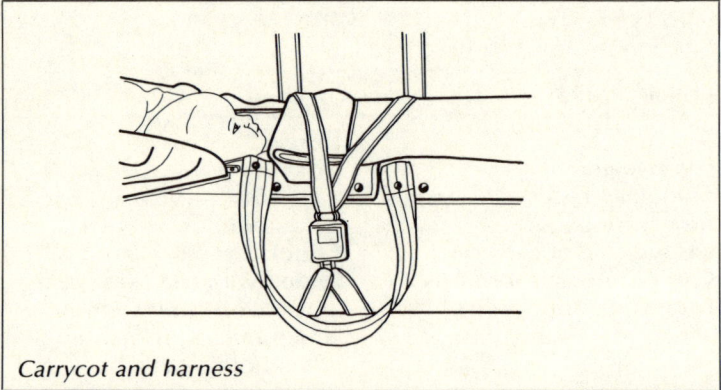

Carrycot and harness

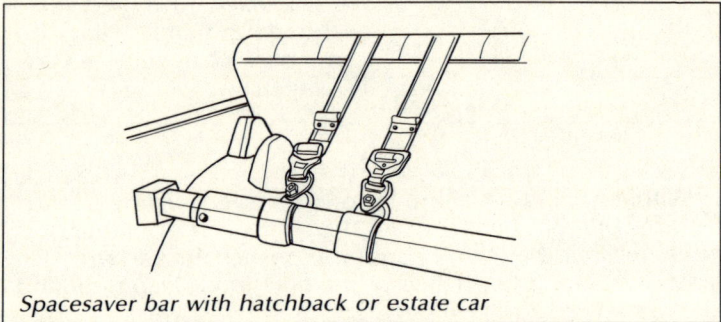

Spacesaver bar with hatchback or estate car

Choose a substantial carrycot and fit a suitable safety harness to hold it in place. Always use the carrycot cover, as otherwise the baby can be thrown out between the straps.

A rear-facing baby seat can be held in place with an adult seat belt. They are very convenient as they can be used in any car, though this may mean relegating an adult passenger to the back seat. This type of seat can also be used as a general seat around the house and when out visiting.

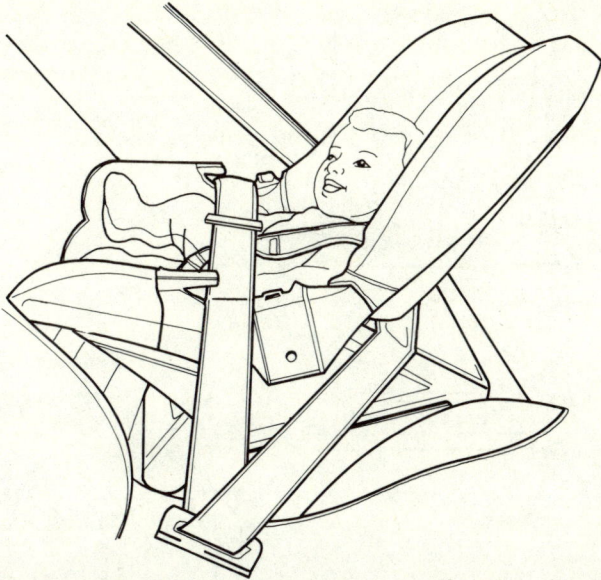

Rear-facing baby seat

From about six to eight months the baby can be moved into a car seat. These can be used with a safety harness fixing kit or some can be used with a car seat belt. Remember when choosing the carrycot that you are likely to have to buy the same brand of car seat if you want to use the same base fixing kit. So look at car seats when you choose the carrycot restraint. In an estate car the fixing kit can take up a fair amount of space. The straps need fixing down to the floor or an estate car bar needs to be fixed across the back to take the seat belts. Either way this takes up quite a lot of the available space. Two-point fixing seats are a better option here, or choose seats that can be used with a rear seat belt.

Any parent starting from scratch will find that the simplest option for safety in the car will be to fit a rear seat belt and then opt for a baby seat for the first nine months or so. Then swop to a child's seat that can be used with a seat belt. This also allows you to use both types of seat in other people's cars.

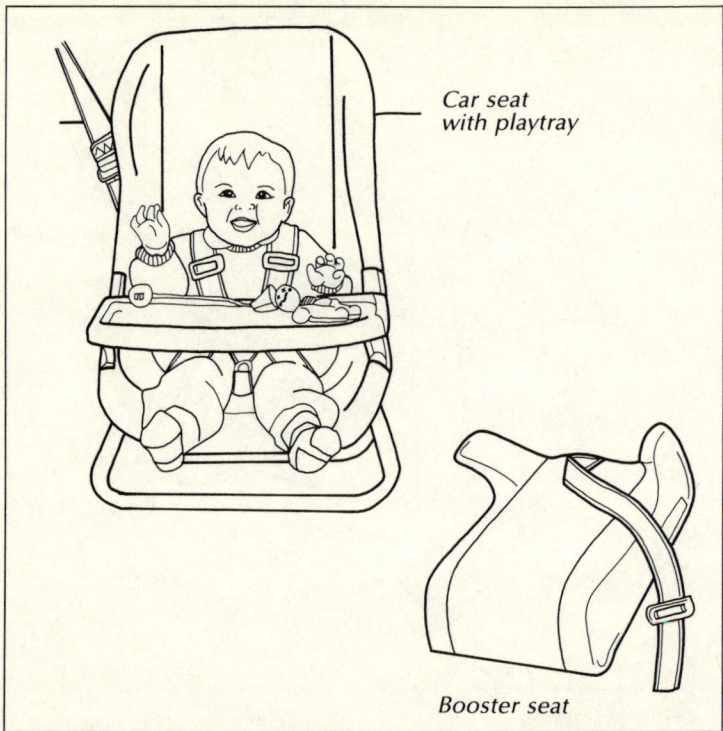

Car seat
with playtray

Booster seat

Reclining seats are more expensive to buy but do allow a sleepy baby to travel comfortably. For any family who undertakes long journeys, the extra cost is well worthwhile. Compare seats, though, as some recline far more than others. Check too how easily the cover removes for washing since drinks and food are often spilt in the car seat.

At about three to four years old, children can move on to free-standing seats and boosters with a seat belt, so you should be able to pass the child's seat on to younger brothers and sisters. Twin car seats are available, though hard to track down. They take up less room than individual seats fitted side by side, but don't recline.

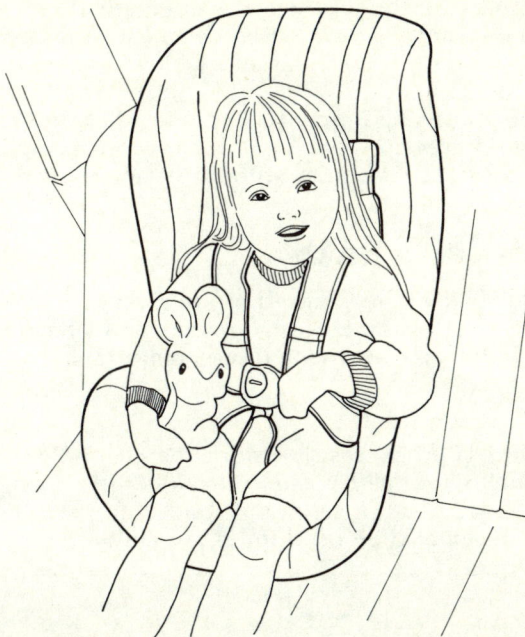

Basic car seat

TRAVEL TIPS

1. Keep journeys short, and do long journeys in short hops. It does take longer but keeps tempers cool.
2. Babies usually sleep, but as they grow older they stay awake for longer in the car. A playtray fitted to the seat with some toys on helps. So too does an adult sitting in the back to keep them company.
3. Music tapes can while away the time. For older children action rhymes and favourite stories help.
4. Take plenty of water to drink in a beaker cup.
5. Keep the car well ventilated.
6. Take a wet flannel in a plastic bag for hand and face washing.
7. Small titbits of food will help keep boredom at bay. Choose foods unlikely to make them sick or messy. Sticks of cheddar cheese, small packets of raisins, little

cheesy biscuits, wedges of apple are ideal.

8. Make breaks in the journey very energetic. Walk in the fresh air and play games rather than just sit in the car.
9. Dress your baby in loose comfortable clothes for travelling.
10. Fit an extra driving mirror (cheap ones that stick on the front windscreen are available in car shops). Angle it so that you can see the baby without having to turn round.

BABIES IN ARMS

Many babies enjoy being carried around, but it is surprising how quickly they become heavy. A sling, and later on a backpack, helps make carrying more comfortable.

SLINGS

Slings vary from pretty basic versions that just hold the baby in roughly the right position, to rather grand affairs that snuggle the baby close to your body and keep him warm. These can also be used for larger children. They

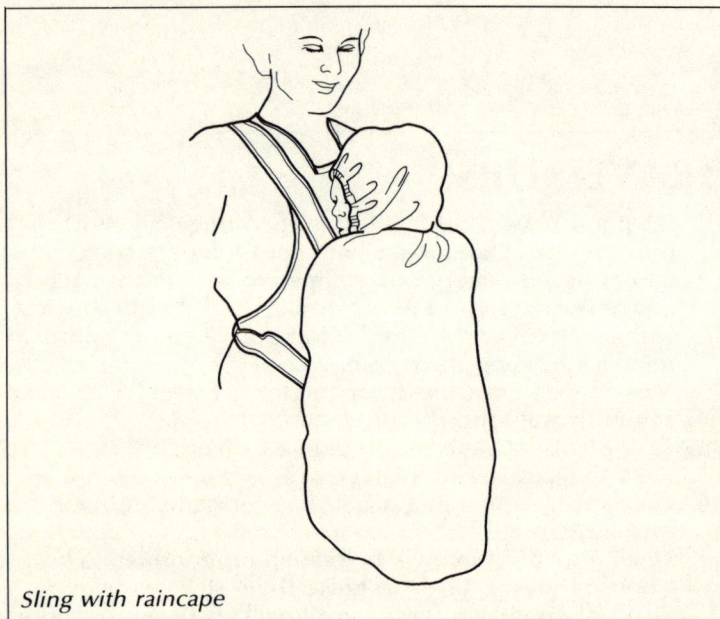

Sling with raincape

have tucks to undo as your baby grows and can be fitted on the adult's back.

New born babies need head support, so choose a sling that holds the head well. Some have clip-on head supports. The most important aspect is how easy the sling is to get on and off. Some tend to need two people to use them. The easiest type allows you to put the sling half on, slide the baby in and then tighten up the sling. Try it out in the shop before choosing. Raincapes are available for some slings to help keep the baby dry and warm.

Only use the sling for short periods as it can strain your back carrying a baby for prolonged periods. Side slings are for older babies (about six months plus) who can be carried on the hip.

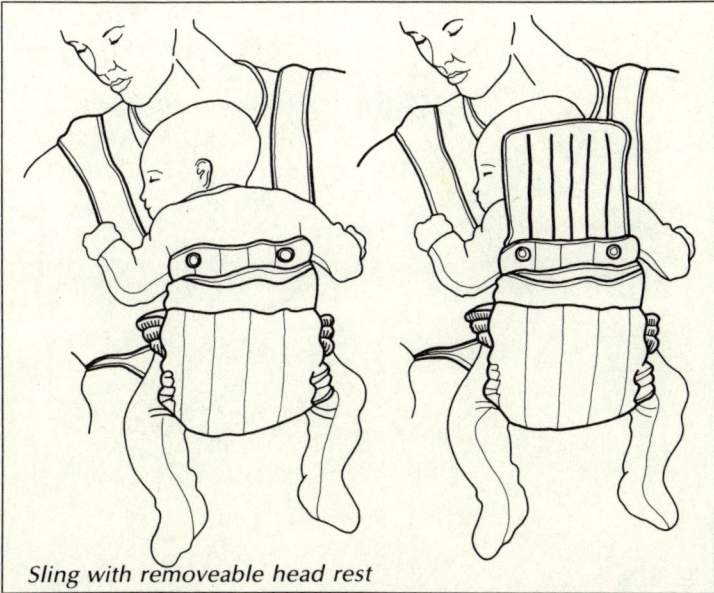

Sling with removeable head rest

BACKPACKS

Backpacks can be used once the baby is sitting well at around six to eight months. They allow you to carry the baby on your back, which is easier with bigger, heavier children. Most have a hip strap, which when tightly done up keeps the frame from bouncing around. It also transfers most of the weight onto your hips, rather than your shoulders. Some backpacks have sunshades, and others have pockets under the seat to take a purse or other small items. Do check that the frame will stand with the baby in it. It should not be used as a seat, but if it will stand firmly it makes getting it on and off much easier.

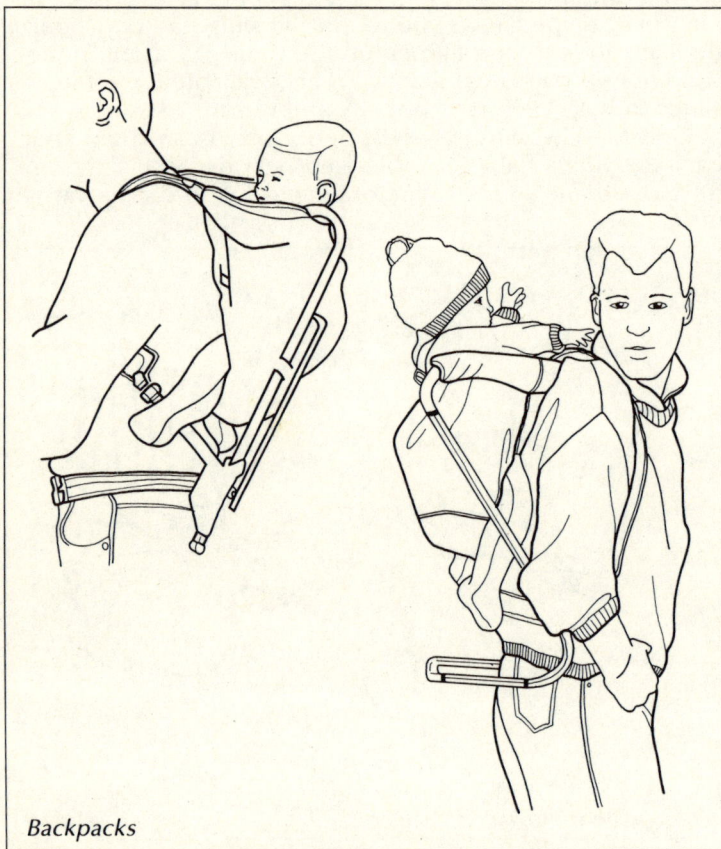

Backpacks

Backpacks are ideal for parents who are keen walkers, as they can be taken where no pushchair can follow.
However, they are also useful when shopping, as the baby is high up and can see around. The parent doesn't have to worry about manoeuvring a pushchair around the Christmas crowds either, but do be careful when you turn round!

BABY CHAIRS, HIGH CHAIRS AND TRAVELLING SEATS

BABY CHAIRS

From around four weeks, babies quite like to sit up and watch what is happening around them. It makes life a little easier as you can fold washing or do the housework around the baby. The simplest baby chairs are fabric stretched over a metal frame. These bounce easily and by around three months many babies find that kicking their legs makes them bounce up and down. Then they will often sit for

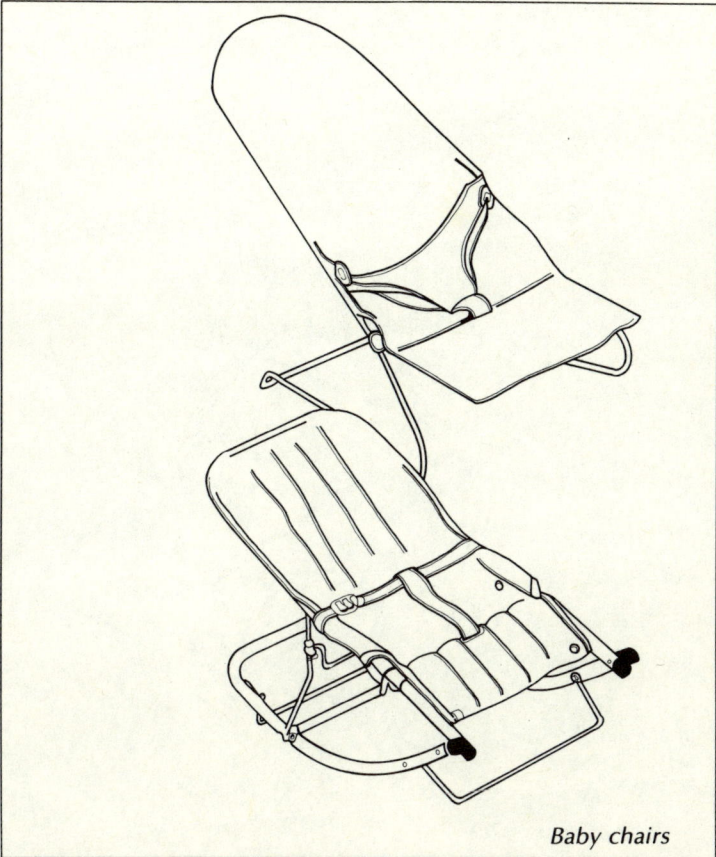

Baby chairs

quite long periods. Toys to fit across the front of this type of chair are also available. The frame folds easily, so that the chair can go flat in the car, and the fabric cover can be removed for washing. Putting the cover back on is always a bit of a puzzle though!

More rigid baby chairs usually have a couple of positions, so that small babies can be reclined and older ones sat upright. They often have padded seat covers which remove for washing. While undoubtedly smart to look at, they are larger than the simple chair and will not pack away as easily. However, they can be used for longer and will usually take a baby up to around a year. The bouncy chairs are outgrown as soon as the baby can lean forward as they tip over quite easily.

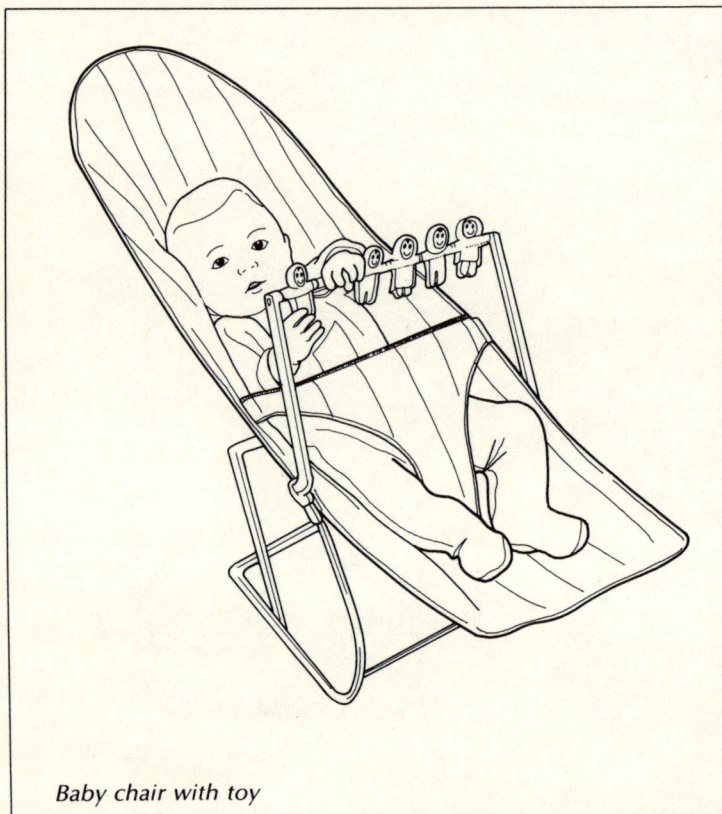

Baby chair with toy

HIGH CHAIRS

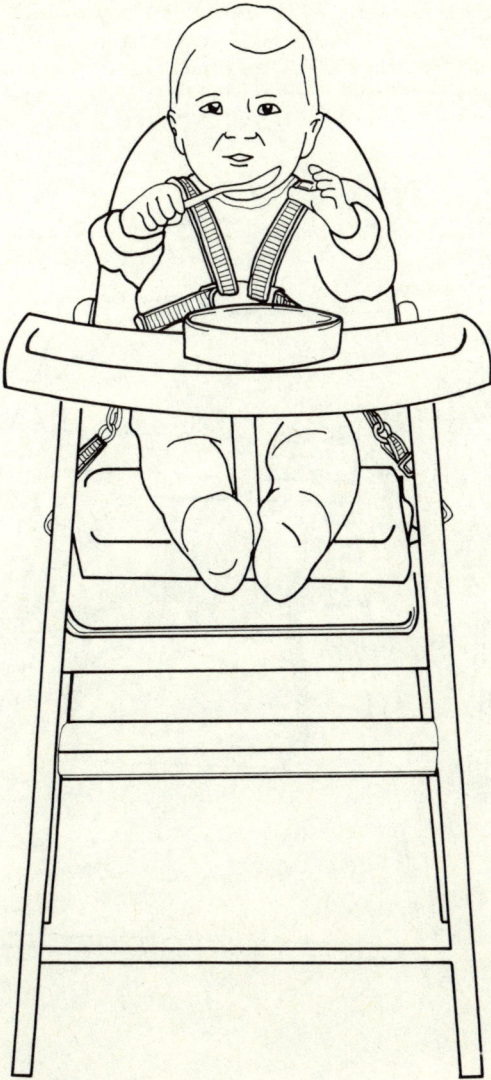

Large high chair

At around six to eight months most babies are sitting up well and eating some solid foods, so a high chair becomes a necessity. It is also useful for your baby to sit and play in when you are cooking as he can be near you but safely out of the way of hot pans. In fact, most families find they go on using a high chair until the child is around two years

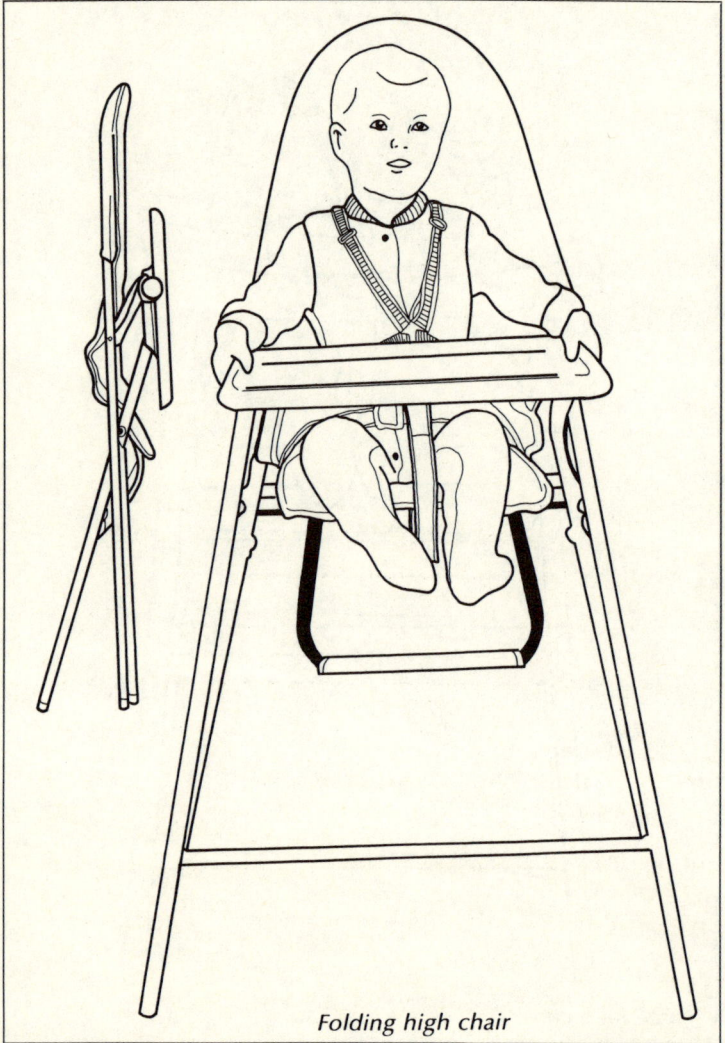

Folding high chair

old. So avoid the temptation to buy a very small chair as you may well have to buy a larger one later. Instead, prop a small baby up with a cushion to fill the space between the seat and the tray.

Stability is very important, particularly on kitchen floors which are often tiled and can be slippery. A wide base helps here. Beware of high chairs with castors: one kick against the table leg and the high chair can go right across the kitchen. In a small kitchen, a folding high chair can save space problems. It is also very useful when going out visiting as it will fit in the back of the car. The high chair

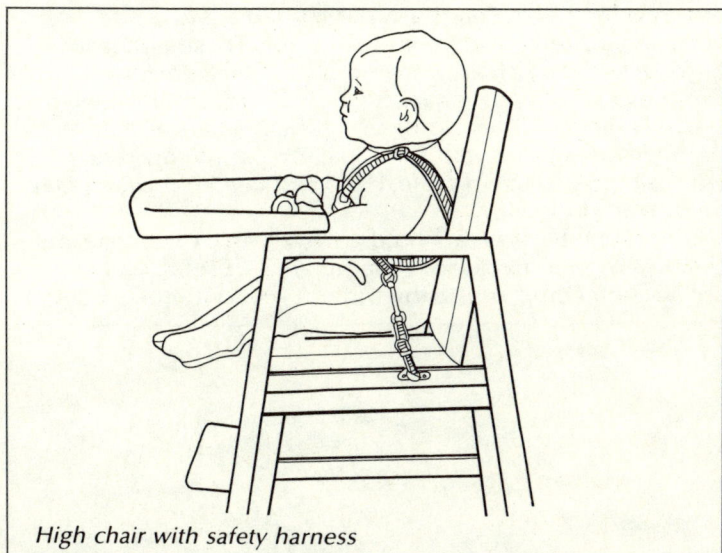

High chair with safety harness

tray needs to be easy to clean. Some can be removed for a once-a-week scrub in the sink. Raised edges to the tray prevent a small child accidentally knocking food off, and make it harder for an older child to do the same deliberately! Fabric seats look pretty and are comfortable, but need more care and attention than wipe-clean ones.

Many high chairs can fold or separate to make a low chair and table. These are useful for playing and for older children to sit and eat at. Check that the seat is close enough to the table, or that it will tuck under. Most children like to sit up close to the table, and this minimises spills. On some high chairs the seat and table, once folded down into a low chair, are in a fixed position and the child has to perch on the edge of the seat in order to use the table.

Always use a harness to hold the baby in the chair. This prevents an active baby climbing out or standing up in the chair. Leave the harness fixed to the chair and just slide the baby in and out, then do up the strap.

TRAVELLING SEATS

Between the ages of around nine months and two years a high chairs does make mealtimes much easier. Often when out travelling high chairs are not available and a portable chair of your own can be a great boon. These either fix onto an ordinary chair or clamp onto a table. Some can be used instead of an ordinary high chair and are ideal where space is limited. They do need a robust chair or table to fix to, and of course if your baby is eating at the main table you will have to avoid tablecloths and keep china and glass items out of the way.

The fabric tie-on seats hold a baby firmly on a chair but don't raise him up to table top height — useful while you are spoonfeeding your baby but not ideal when he wants to

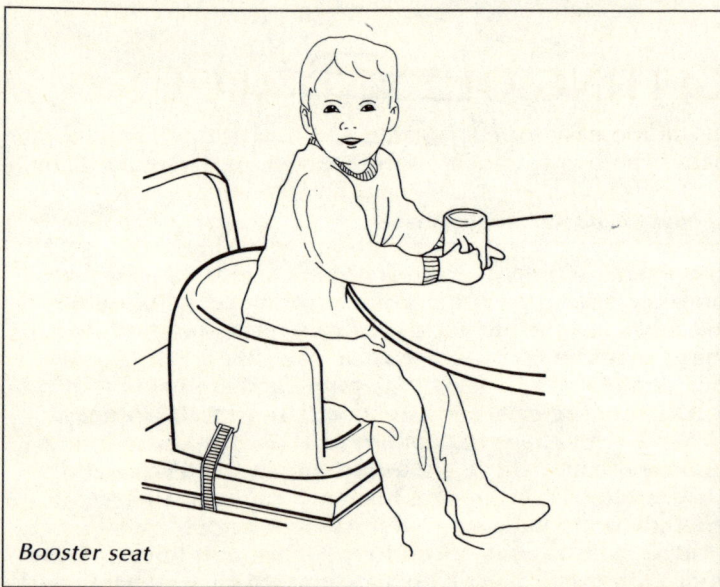

Booster seat

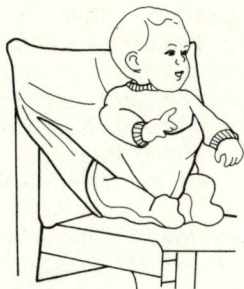

Fabric tie-on seat

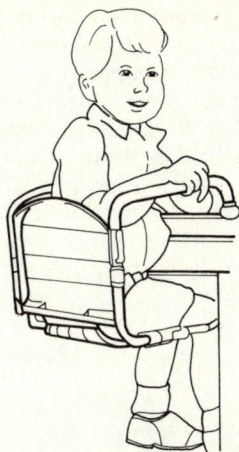

Clamp-on seat

feed himself. Since they are made of fabric they are quite cheap to buy or can easily be made.

The clamp-on chairs are rather more expensive but robust enough to use as a substitute high chair.

GETTING OUT AND ABOUT

It's all too easy to feel isolated and housebound with a baby. There is so much effort involved in getting the baby ready to go out, and few enough places where a tiny baby is really welcome that it can be easier to stay in. However, a new mother's best friends are other mothers. They understand the frustration of not being able to get into shops or up escalators, of cafés that put out signs saying 'no pushchairs allowed', and of only ever being able to take the pram as far as you can walk since it won't fit on the bus.

Often the mothers you meet at antenatal classes or clinics become firm friends. If not, ask your health visitor if there are any other new mothers nearby, or if there are any coffee mornings you can go to. In some areas there are postnatal exercise classes too. Churches often have young wives groups or new mother groups you can attend. Try your local mother and toddler group. Many welcome new mothers, even when their babies are tiny, and often they have nearly new sales as well. Try your local branch of the NCT (page 154 or local telephone directory). Many have neighbourhood support groups that meet regularly for coffee, or to go swimming or on picnics etc. Meet-a-Mum (page 153 or local telephone directory) is another organisation that helps support new mothers. Many adult education centres have crèches so you can spend some time learning a new skill as well as meeting other mothers.

If none of these things appeals or there are none in your area, try putting a card in a shop window inviting other mothers to contact you. Several of the major magazines for new parents run columns for people to advertise and exchange information. You could always run a coffee afternoon yourself. Arrange one for a charity, advertise it locally and stress that new mothers with babies are particularly welcome. You may well find there are several mothers in the same area, all feeling equally isolated.

4 BABIES ON THE MOVE

By around nine months many babies are crawling or shuffling along on their bottoms. At around a year or soon after most babies are beginning to walk. These stages vary from child to child, of course, so don't panic just because your neighbour's child is a week or two ahead of yours!

Once babies are mobile they begin to take over your household. They will crawl over and empty the litter bin, reach up and pull over plants and even tip a hot cup of coffee over themselves if you leave it on a low table. So child-proof your house before this stage of exploration. Go round and move everything up, well out of reach. Re-arrange furniture to protect more precious objects and fit stair gates and socket covers. Try going round on your hands and knees and move anything potentially fascinating to a baby.

PLAYPENS

In some households a playpen is vital to protect the child from potentially dangerous things that cannot be moved, e.g. split level rooms or several pets, or even older brothers and sisters! Many parents find them helpful for short periods when they know they will be distracted, such as while ironing or while going to answer the door. However, playpens are easily abused. Newly mobile children are naturally inquisitive and enjoy exploring the house. In many ways this is an easy phase if you make the effort to make the house safe. Leave one cupboard in the kitchen full of soft plastic boxes, spoons and empty cartons, and your ten-month-old will happily spend half the afternoon emptying it out and climbing in himself. So resist the temptation to abandon the baby to the playpen if possible and instead help him to be safely mobile.

Wooden playpens are the traditional type, but playpens with fine mesh sides are also available. Either type needs to have a well-padded floor, and removable wipe-clean

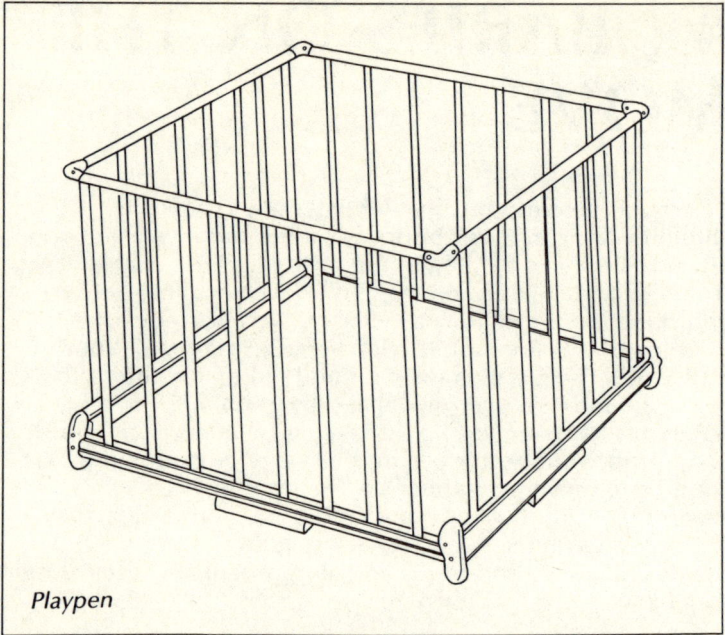

Playpen

padded mats are available. Some come with them as standard, with others they are an optional extra. The mesh type do need to have a really fine mesh, otherwise the baby's fingers or buttons can become entangled. This type do tend to develop holes in the mesh sides as they wear. A well-padded rim is essential to prevent the child bumping his chin when he stands holding onto the sides. Check how safe the outside of the playpen is too, in case older children are playing nearby; look for protruding screws or nuts or folding sections that could catch a child's fingers.

Wooden playpens need to be smoothly finished all over so no splinters will appear. This type generally cost a little more than the mesh type but will last longer. You may even find yourself using one for your own grandchildren in years to come. They are a good secondhand buy as well.

Both types of playpen can be used in the garden too, and are useful when your child is crawling and it's too wet to let him get out on the grass. Almost all have raised floors which ensure the child stays warm and dry even on a damp surface.

BOUNCERS

Long before your baby can crawl he may well enjoy making himself mobile in a bouncer. These consist of a fabric seat which ties around the baby's body and hangs from a spring. Suspended from a hook in a doorway, or on a special stand, the baby can bounce around and enjoy the sensation of moving his own body for short periods. They are useful from when your baby has firm head control until he weighs too much for the bouncer. Usually the limit is around 14kg/30 lb. They are designed to be used for short periods, say twenty minutes or so at a time. Used with a clamp instead of a hook they will fit over most doorways so

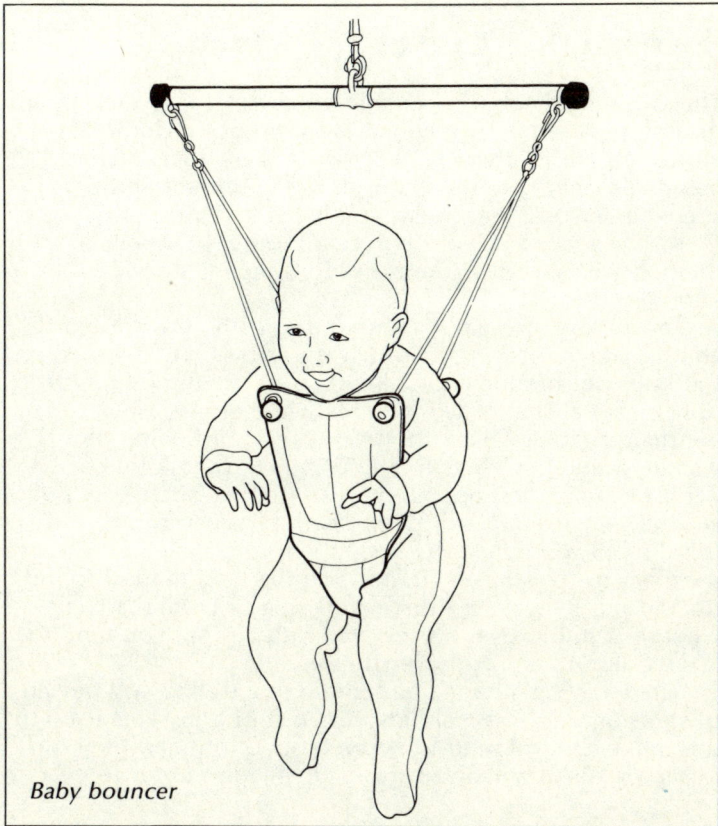

Baby bouncer

you can move the baby around with you while you clean the bath, cook a meal or write your first novel!

Never leave a baby unattended in a bouncer, and always double check the fastenings. Arrange the bouncer so that the baby's feet just touch the floor. This allows him to bounce up and down without taking his own weight. Beware of visiting children or pets pushing past him to get through the doorway. Older children have been known to use the bouncer as a lifesize catapult for their smaller siblings or to spin them round mercilessly. We tied some little bells and plastic spoons on the bar of the bouncer so that it made a noise as the baby bounced. The baby made a noise as he bounced too, so it was definitely a game for short periods only, but great fun for all concerned.

BABY WALKERS

These wheeled supports enable a baby to get around in an upright position before he can walk properly. Some have fabric seats and others plastic trays to take toys. Many babies do enjoy the sensation of being upright and able to see what is going on. Most rapidly learn to propel themselves forward with their feet. Some, however, hate them, so do try out a friend's before buying one for your baby.

Check how the seat is fixed underneath. You should be able to adjust the height so that the baby's feet just rest on the floor but he does not take his own weight. Some can only be set at one or two heights while others are multi-adjustable. Check too the method of folding the walker. Some have legs that fold in half, others fold vertically and some operate like an ironing board. Try out several. The ironing board type is the easiest to fold and unfold and you adjust the height with the same mechanism. This means in practice that you tend to fold it up and put it away, say under the sofa or behind a chair when it is not in use. If they are fiddly to fold you tend to leave them up and trip over them.

Avoid leaving a baby unattended in a walker and beware of steps and door thresholds. Once your baby gets used to the walker he will tend to zoom around in it and they can tip up by rushing at an obstacle at speed in order to get over it.

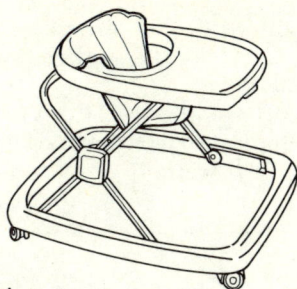

Baby walker with tray

Again these are designed to be used for short periods only. There is some argument over the use of baby walkers. Some experts think they actually inhibit a baby from walking properly as he becomes used to relying on the walker. It may be worth hiring or borrowing a walker, or even buying a secondhand one, as the time span for which they are used is quite short.

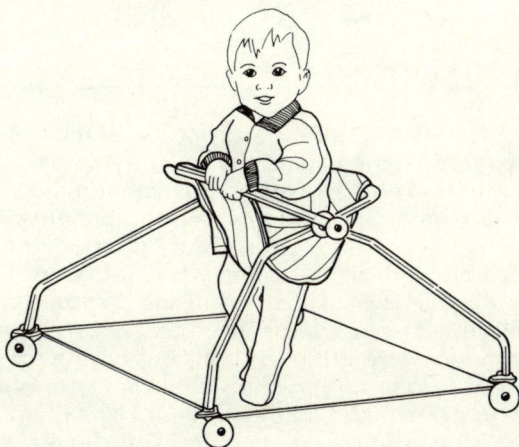

Baby walker

TOYS

Play is a very important part of a baby's life. Through play your baby learns about the world, and develops his muscles and co-ordination.

Toys don't have to come in boxes from toy shops. To a child almost everything is a toy. The very best sorts of toys are other people who will respond to him and help amuse him.

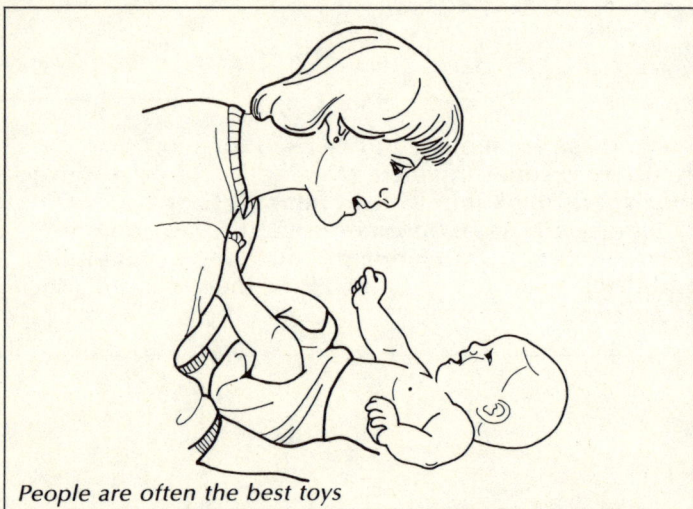

People are often the best toys

Newborn babies will follow your face with their eyes, try to imitate your movements and the noises you make to them. By around five to six weeks movement, colour and shape become important, and mobiles and pictures hung above your baby's cot are a good idea. Of course you may want to decorate your baby's room with mobiles well before this stage anyway. When choosing a mobile check what it looks like from underneath. Many are very pretty for adults who look from the side on, but boring for the baby who looks from underneath. Pin a variety of objects onto a cotton parasol and fix this to the baby's pram or cot. Change the items round occassionally. You can make up your own mobile by hanging a variety of objects onto a coat hanger. Make sure they are all firmly fixed on and hang the hanger above the cot where it cannot be reached

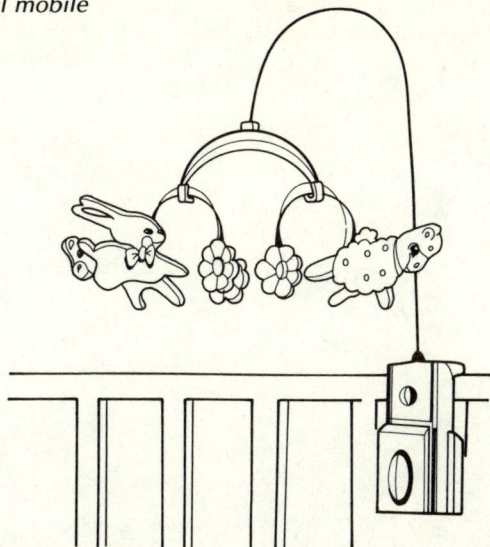

Musical mobile

if your baby is big enough to sit up. Try hanging coloured plastic spoons, shapes cut from felt or stiff card, a small toy such as a rattle, a coloured feather or a plastic cup upside down etc. Change the items every now and then too. Place the pram under a tree or near the washing in the garden so the movement attracts the baby.

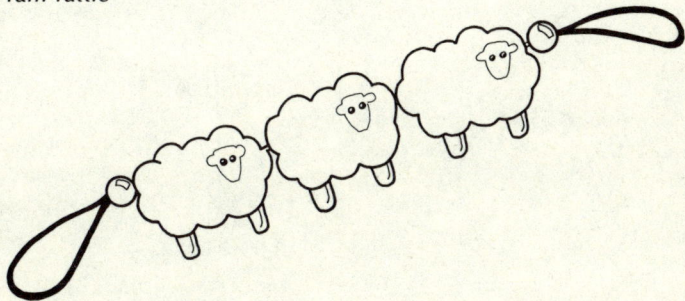

Pram rattle

As soon as your baby can reach out to hold things, rattles and activity toys become important. There is a wide variety of rattles on the market. A first rattle needs to be narrow enough for a baby to hold easily, and interesting

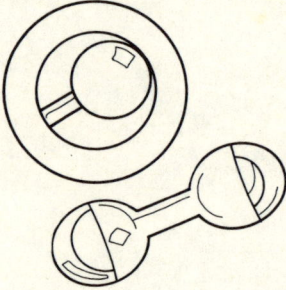

Rattles

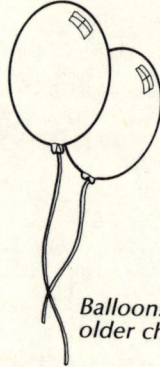

Balloons for older children

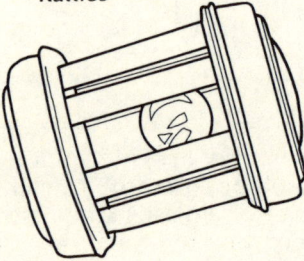

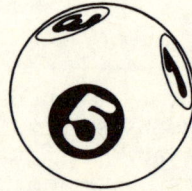

Musical ball

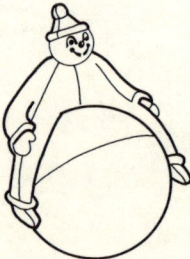

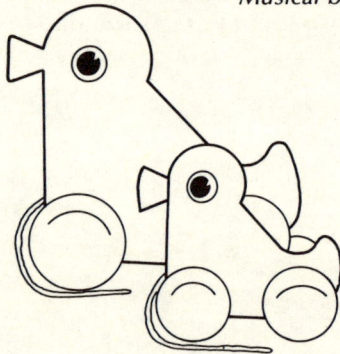

Pullalong and pushalong toys

enough for him to want to hold it. So bright colours and interesting shapes to feel matter as much as a good noise. Check that the rattle has no sharp edges or places for fingers to become trapped.

Activity toys can be fixed to the side of the cot or used on the floor. They have a variety of toys included in them. This makes them very versatile and you may well find that the toy goes on being used throughout the first year and longer. At first your baby will smile into the little mirror and accidentally knock a lever or two. Then as he grows stronger and more co-ordinated he will be able to play with other parts of the activity toy. So although this type of toy may seem expensive at first it does generally give plenty of play value over a long period. They can also be bought secondhand.

Once your baby can sit up he may well enjoy games of putting things inside each other. Stacking rings and beakers or barrels are ideal at this stage. You can supply a range of suitable containers from the kitchen, and save yoghurt and margarine tubs for playing with. Later, sorting becomes a favourite game and cotton reels or plastic spoons are useful for this stage. Keep a collection of suitable objects in a large plastic tub.

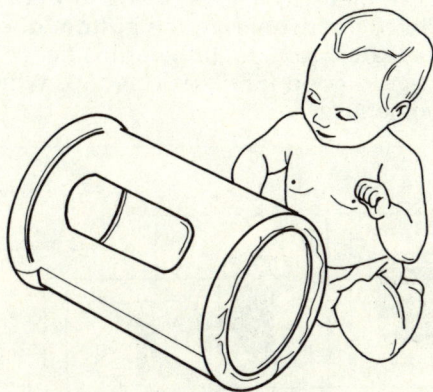

See-through pushalong toy

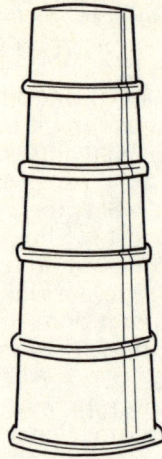
Stacking cups

In the garden in summer, water play is great fun. A large washing up bowl or a small paddling pool with plenty of warm water will keep him occupied for long periods. Play with him and don't leave him unattended near water, even small amounts. Give him plastic jugs or yoghurt pots for pouring water. Pierce a few holes in the bottom of one tub so he can feel the water sprinkle out over his hands. A large natural sponge is good for squeezing too. Wind-up toys that swim will amuse.

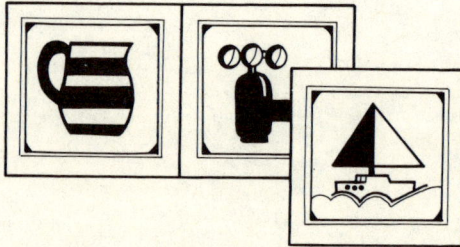
Board books

Games with adults are great fun. Peekaboo is popular from around five or six months until they are three or four years old. Try showing your baby a toy and then hiding it under a scarf or blanket. At first he will not be able to understand that the toy is under the blanket, but gradually he will realise and join in the game of searching for the toy. Then try hiding a small toy in your hand and let him open up your finger to look for it. Later you can hide things behind your back.

Activity games are good fun for everyone. Try cycling your baby's legs in the air while he is lying on his back on the floor. Or lay him flat and move his arms up and down. Keep your face close to his while you do it. Try blowing raspberries on his tummy or kissing his bare skin. Pretending to nibble his fingers usually tickles a bit and can be a great game. Let him lie on your tummy while you lie flat on your back on the floor and bounce him up and down gently. Or lie on your back with your legs raised up and lie him along them. Then lift your legs up and down so he rides with them. The possibilities are endless if you can overcome your adult inhibitions and actually get down on the floor and play with your baby. Play gently at first and avoid sessions when your baby is tired, hungry or has just been fed.

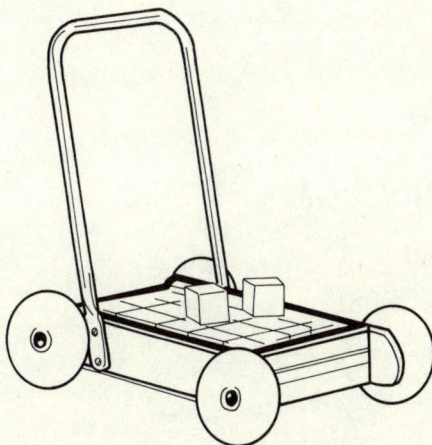

Trolley with bricks

STAGES OF PLAY

AGE	TOYS
Six weeks	Mobiles suspended over cot. Adults talking to baby; close eye to eye contact.
Four-five months	Small rattles to hold and move. Activity centre in cot. Watching adults and other children while sitting in a bouncy chair.
Six-eight months	Stacking and sorting toys. Large beach ball or inflatable toy for attempting to push or for rolling between parent and baby. Toys which make a noise when pushed or hit. Try adding some rice grains to an empty custard tin. Seal the lid well and then roll across the floor. Board books.

Ride-on toy

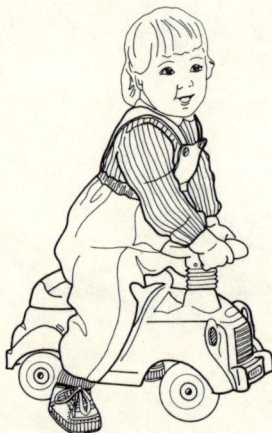

AGE	TOYS
Nine-twelve months	Sturdy pushalong toys which help with walking.
	Toys with strings on that can easily be pulled towards the child while he is sitting.
	A large balloon on a string (but supervise well in case it bursts).
	Posting toys. A nappy box with a hole cut in for posting letters, or a small plastic toy with shaped slots for posting.
	Books with activity songs.
	A scrapbook with pictures cut from magazines.
	A sturdy bag for playing shopping or for squirrelling away favourite toys.
	Old hats for dressing up.

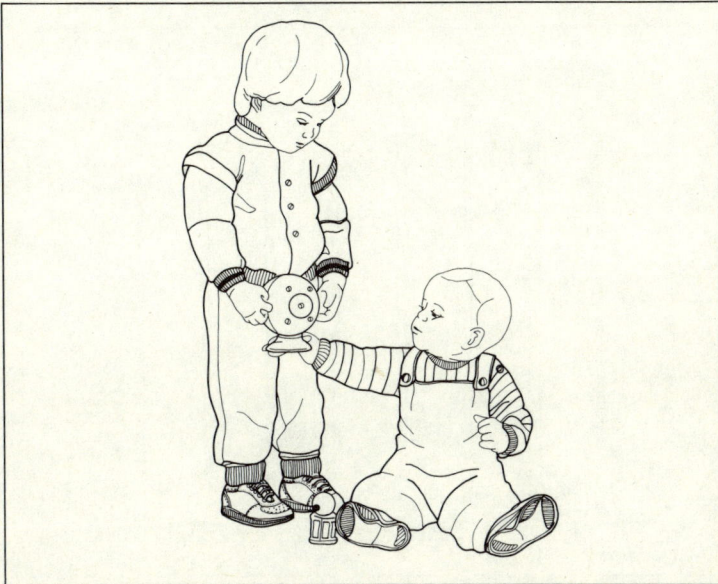

SAFETY

Safety equipment is an essential investment in any home with small children. It is important that any safety device you buy is robust and easy to use. If it takes time to fiddle putting up the stair gate or using the cupboard lock there will come a day when you don't bother, and that will be the time when an accident will occur. So compare what's available and look at friends' houses and see what works and what doesn't. Here are details of most household safety devices.

STAIR GATES

As soon as your baby is mobile and until he is three or four years old, stair gates will be a vital part of your household. The choice is for fixed or moveable stair gates. Fixed ones are easy to use since they open like a door or fold up onto a wall. Moveable ones take longer to use, since you need to fit them and remove them each time, but they can be used on doorways as well as on the stairs. This is useful when you need to keep your child out of one room for a short time, such as when decorating, when cooking or

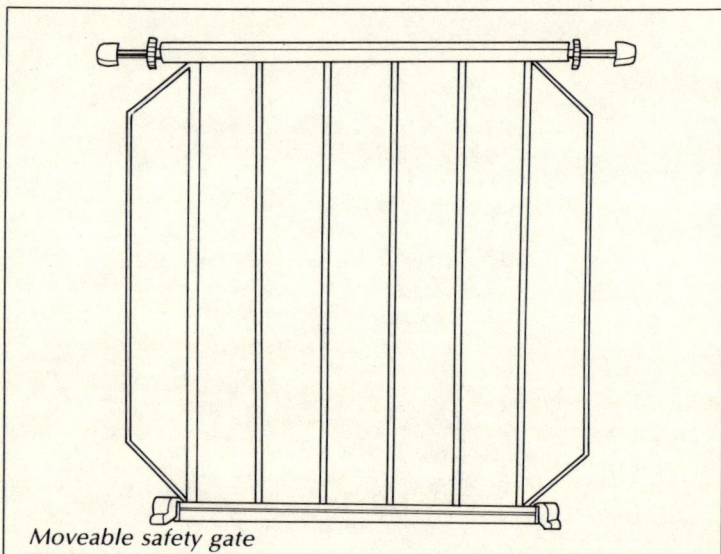

Moveable safety gate

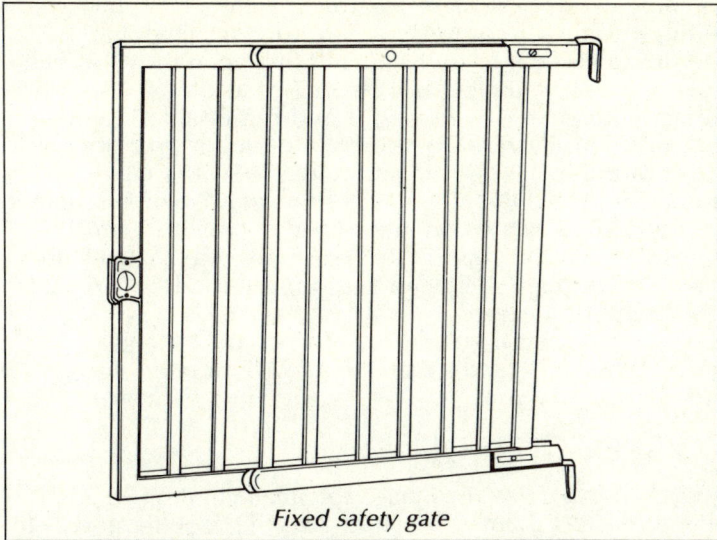

Fixed safety gate

when getting ready for a birthday party. He can still see you through the stair gate, and you can keep an eye on him while you work.

Stair gates at the top and bottom of the stairs are ideal. Or use one moveable gate and fit it according to where you are playing/working. So most of the time it will need to be at the bottom of the stairs, but when you go upstairs to make the beds, have a bath, or at night, you will need to fit it at the top of the stairs.

Look for stair gates built to British Standards. This governs the width of the gaps and how tall they are as well as the design. Stairgates can cause accidents simply because so many adults attempt to hop over them rather than undo them! Many families find it's worth fitting the more expensive opening-style stair gate at the bottom of the stairs where it's used most often. A cheaper moveable one can be used at the top. Extension pieces are available on some stair gates for extra wide stairways and corridors.

FIREGUARDS

All fires should be guarded when there are children in the house. As well as preventing a child falling onto a fire or catching his clothes alight, guards prevent a child throwing things into the fire or pushing furniture close enough to the fire to cause it to burn. It's not just open fires that need guarding. Gas and electric fires are just as dangerous. A nursery fire guard is very strong and can be fitted to the wall or fireplace so that a baby cannot pull it over or move it out of the way. They are adjustable so will fit most fireplaces. Avoid the temptation to hang washing on them to dry, and be aware that many children will post small items through the guard. Our house rule was that any item that went through the guard was not returned, which made it a very boring game.

There are special guards available for portable gas heaters too, and guards that can be wall mounted for gas fires set up on a wall.

COOKER GUARDS

A kitchen is a dangerous place for small children so it is vital to protect them as much as possible. Cooker guards fit over the hob of a free-standing cooker and prevent pans toppling over. They are simple and easy to fit and remain on the cooker all the time, except for occasional cleaning. Special guards are available for split level hobs. Even with a guard in place make an effort to get in the habit of using the hotplate or gas burners at the back of the hob so that pans cannot be reached by a toddler. Also, always turn the pan handles away from the front of the worktop.

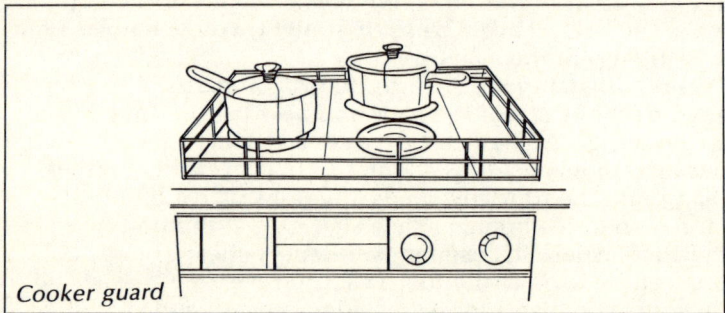

Cooker guard

The rest of the cooker is harder to make childproof. The exterior of the oven can become very hot when in use. A child falling against it could be burned, especially if there are metal trims or handles. It does vary from brand to brand.

Many British cookers have extra insulation while some cheap imported cookers have very little. So be aware of the danger. Low-level grills are fascinating to toddlers and crawling children. The flap down door is often a good height to pull themselves up on, and the glowing red elements inside attract them. My own son reached in and touched the element one lunchtime while waiting for his fish fingers to be cooked. He simply did not realise they would be hot and ended up with very badly burned fingers. His other trick was to post small toys into the grill. If I forgot to check we ended up with melted plastic all over the grill pan and a pretty awful smell throughout the house!

CUPBOARD AND DOOR LOCKS AND SOCKET COVERS

These are very simple gadgets that can be fitted inside most cupboards or drawers. They automatically close when you close the cupboard; to open them you usually have to put your finger inside and release them as you open the door.

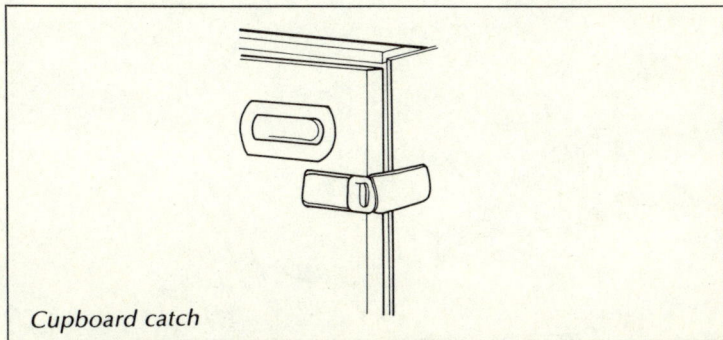

Cupboard catch

Children do eventually work out how to open them (usually by around four or five years), but by the time they have the co-ordination and intelligence to do so they are sensible enough to be taught why they should not touch whatever is inside. Special locks for refrigerators are also available, and there is even a 'loo lock'. This holds the seat and lid onto the toilet bowl. It may seem superfluous but if you have ever seen a teddy bear or spare toilet roll posted down the loo and the chain pulled repeatedly on top you will appreciate the mess involved.

Socket covers are also available which prevent tiny fingers or other things being pushed into electricity sockets.

WALKING REINS

These were very popular a couple of generations ago and are now very much underestimated. They do make it easy to hang on to a child who wants to walk but has no traffic sense. They also help a newly walking child to be steady on his feet as you can take his weight if he falls. Most children enjoy them if they are allowed to play games like being a horse in them. The reins need to be strong and robust, and easy to clip on and off. Check that the fastening will not

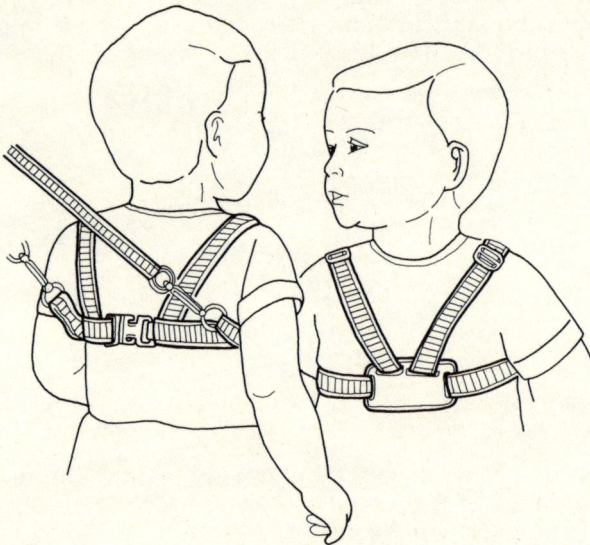

Walking reins

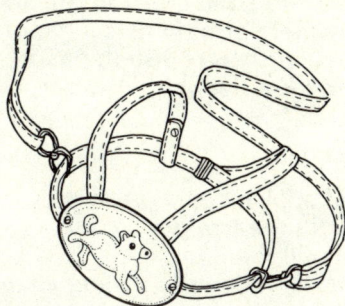

Leather walking reins

work loose while walking and that they do up at the back where the child cannot fiddle with them. The walking lead unclips so that the harness can be used in a high chair. Clips that remain on the harness section (rather than on the lead) allow it to be used to secure a child in a supermarket trolley too. Make sure the harness can be washed or scrubbed, as it will soon get dirty when being used in a high chair. It's a good policy to leave the harness in place

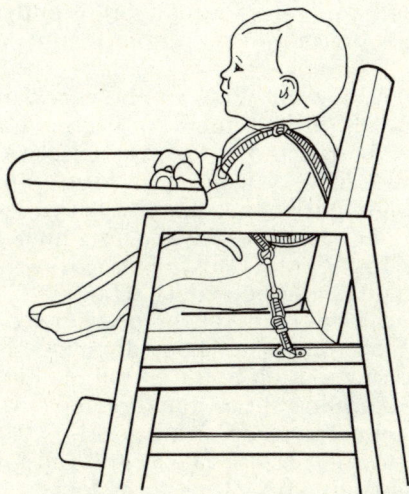

Safety harness in high chair

on the highchair and simply slide the child in and out. That way it will always be to hand and you will always use it. If you leave it somewhere else there is a temptation to put your baby in the chair then realise the harness is missing and go off to look for it, leaving the baby unrestrained.

SAFETY TIPS

1. Keep leads on appliances short so they don't dangle over the edge of the worktop where a small child could reach up and pull them off.
2. Avoid using tablecloths: the trailing edges tempt a crawling baby to pull himself up on them.
3. Don't leave knives out on the worktop. Fit a magnetic knife rack high on the wall or use a knife block, or put them in a drawer.
4. Freezers can give a nasty burn. Use a 'fridge lock on low-level front-opening freezers.
5. Keep plants and flowers up high, otherwise toddlers will tip them over or uproot them. Trailing plants are often at just the right height for a toddler to pull them over on top of himself.
6. Scissors, pins, needles and coins all need storing out of reach. It's so easy to put them down on the coffee table for a few minutes and forget them. Put a wicker basket on a high shelf and get into the habit of putting sharp or dangerous objects into this rather than just on the table.
7. Glass doors and low windows can be very dangerous. Toddlers may fall through them, or even attempt to walk through them without realising the glass is there. Line with safety film, available from major nursery shops, and highlight with stickers so it's easy to see.
8. Store bleach and cleaning powders in a high cupboard or lock them in the under sink cupboard. Do the same with bathroom cleaning powders etc.
9. Also lock up bubble bath, talcum powder etc. They make a terrible mess if your baby discovers them. My toddler once threw a full bottle of bubble bath down the stairs; the bottle split on the top step and sprayed its contents onto each step as it passed!
10. Dishwasher powder is very caustic and can burn the skin on a child's tongue. Store it in a locked cupboard and only put it in the machine when you are ready to

run the programme.

11. Turn the washing machine and tumble dryer off at the plug when not in use to foil children playing with the controls.

12. Make a habit of putting all plastic bags safely out of the way immediately you unpack things. Keep in a high cupboard. Don't just throw them away in the waste bin where they might be discovered and played with. Put them straight in the dustbin instead.

13. Remove lids from canned foods completely. Drop them inside the empty can and then fill with other rubbish such as potato peelings or screwed-up paper bags. When the lid is only partly removed small fingers can easily be trapped down the side of the can and it is then very hard to remove it without cutting your child's hands badly.

14. Avoid ironing with your child around. That moving flex is a terrible temptation to a baby sitting near your feet. Either iron when your child is asleep or put up a stair gate and iron one side of it while your baby plays on the other side. I know one woman who does her ironing inside the playpen while her children play outside of it!

15. Always try to keep one step ahead of your child. View your house from his level; get down on hands and knees and look at what he can see that might just cause an accident. **Before** he crawls, put in socket covers, fit cupboard locks and stair gates. **Before** he pulls himself up, remove anything which might topple over. **Before** he walks, check what he might just walk into. It's worth the time and effort to make your home as safe as possible.

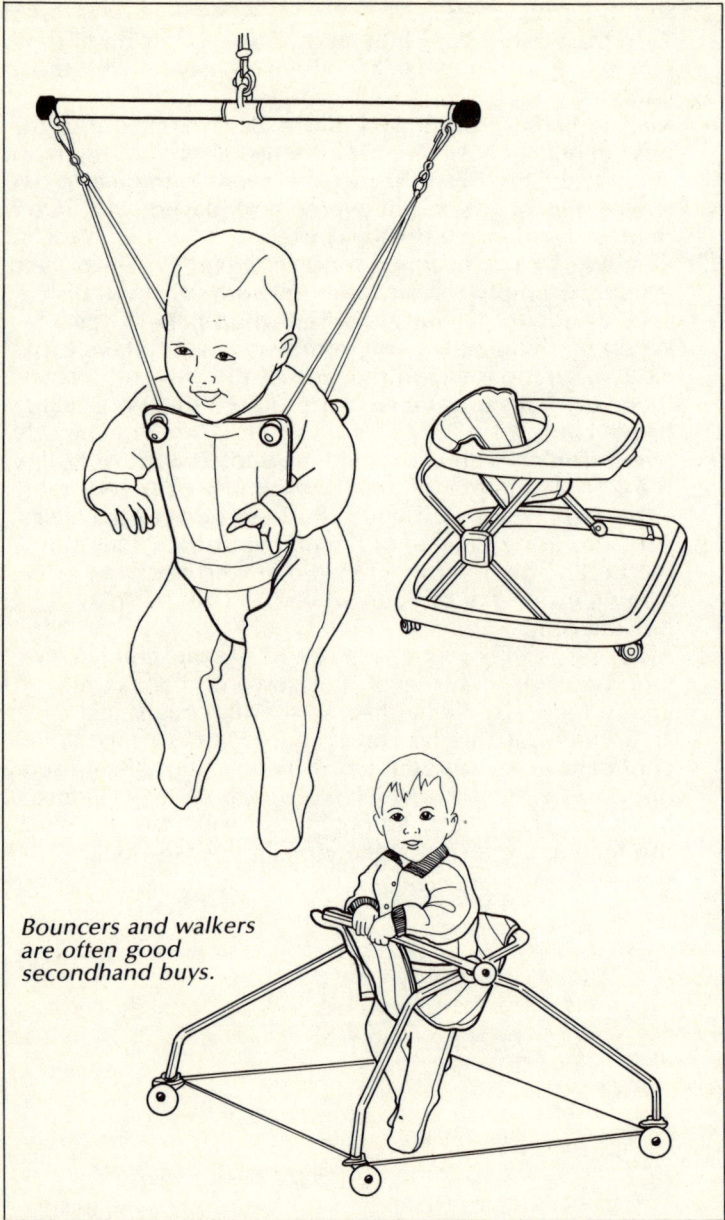

*Bouncers and walkers
are often good
secondhand buys.*

5 BUYING SECONDHAND

Secondhand equipment is often good value. So much baby equipment is only used for short periods that it is outgrown rather than worn out. However, buying anything secondhand has its pitfalls. If the equipment appears unused, ask why; it may simply be that their extra large baby never fitted into the extra small carrycot, or the rapid arrival of a younger sibling means they now need a double buggy rather than a single one. However, it may be that they found the thing they are selling inconvenient, unsuitable or too flimsy, in which case so might you!

WHAT TO BUY

Some things are worth buying secondhand, while others are likely to be a poor buy. Mostly it depends on the amount of wear the item will have had. A pram is usually only used for five or six months so is likely to be in reasonable condition. A buggy tends to be used for two to three years per baby, so after a couple of children it may well be worn out.

Also the condition of the equipment will matter a great deal; it needs to be safe and clean, and the price needs to be reasonable. Compare the price with the cost of the same thing brand new, and with other secondhand versions. Add any extra costs like servicing, repainting or spare parts. Some reductions are well worth having, others are pretty minimal. Also, look closely at the condition. Some things are reasonably easy to repair or replace, like missing screws, while others, like torn linings, are much harder to deal with.

GOOD SECONDHAND BUYS

ITEM	WHAT TO LOOK FOR
Baby baths and stands	Make sure the bath and stand fit well.
	Check that there are no missing screws in the stand, or if there are that you can replace them easily.
	The bath should still be smooth on the inside, so that it is easy to clean. Over-enthusiastic use of a harsh abrasive may have scratched it.
Carrycots/ transporters Prams	Check the condition of the wheels. You may be able to order new ones if they are a major brand, or from a major nursery store.
	Look for chipped paint or rust spots on chrome. Small spots can be touched up, but larger areas are a nuisance. Check the handles on a carrycot are still firmly fixed and not likely to wear. Make sure there are no splits in the hood or lining. Small tears or splits can be mended temporarily using a sticking plaster on the inside, but proper repairs are much harder and really need doing professionally.
	Fold and unfold the chassis yourself and check the locking devices.
	Look for missing screws and knobs; compare with the remaining ones to see if you are likely to be able to match them.
	Finally, check that all the pieces are there; is there a shopping tray, rain cover, sun canopy etc.?

ITEM	WHAT TO LOOK FOR
Baby walkers	Make sure there are no missing wheels, and that the folding mechanism still works smoothly.
	Trays should be smooth and clean.
	Toys fixed to the tray should be complete and not cracked or broken.
Bouncing chairs/baby seats	Most of these have washable seats so they should be clean.
	Chrome bouncing chairs are prone to spots of rust, especially if they have been stored in a damp cellar or garage. Small spots can be dealt with, see pages 125–7 on cleaning baby equipment.
	Check that reclining chairs still work and that fixing points for toys are not broken.
Cots	Look for chipped and flaking paintwork, or woodwork with splinters.
	Check for any rust on the mechanism which drops the sides.
	If it is very old it may have pieces that protrude above the side on which a child's clothes could get hooked. Also the cot bars may be too wide, allowing a child to put his head through. The British Standards recommends a minimum of 2.5 cm/1 inch and a maximum of 6 cm/$2\frac{1}{4}$ ins.
	Look at the mattress; if it is torn or damaged it will be worth buying a new one as long as the cot is a standard size. Make sure the mattress fits well; if it is too small the baby may slip through the side and if it is too large he may climb onto the side of the mattress and hoist himself up and out of the cot. Check that transfers stuck onto the cot are firmly stuck down or can easily be completely removed.

ITEM	WHAT TO LOOK FOR
High chairs	Check for stability.
	Look for missing screws or bolts.
	Paintwork or woodwork should be smooth and free from splinters or flaking paint.
	Trays should be clean and uncracked. Make sure the top surface is smooth; harsh abrasives may have made it rough and it will then be difficult to keep clean.
	If the high chair folds into a low chair and table, try folding it yourself and check there are no cracks, splits or very dirty marks underneath. Fabric and plastic seats can become torn or wear very thin with repeated washing so check this too.
Slings and carriers	**Slings** are only used for a few months so should be a good buy. Most are washable, so they should also be clean.
	Check that any plastic buckles or clips are not broken, and that the headrest (if there is one) still fits well.
	Also, try it on to make sure that it will fit around you. Some straps are rather short for fathers a little on the large side!
	Carriers generally get used for longer than slings but less frequently, so are often a good buy.
	Make sure none of the straps is frayed or worn, and that the fabric seat is not damaged in any way.
	Check that it has a strap that fits around the parents' hips. Once done up this strap moves most of the baby's weight onto the hips, rather than the shoulders. A few old versions were sold without this hip strap, making carrying a toddler much harder.

ITEM	WHAT TO LOOK FOR
Sterilising kits	These are often bought 'just in case' and never used. If they have been used you will have to replace the teats, obviously, but the bottles and all other parts should be able to be re-used since they can be sterilised.
	Discard any cracked or chipped bottles or any that look very old. They are quite cheap to renew anyway.

WHAT NOT TO BUY

Some items of baby equipment are best bought new, unless you know the past history of it. Buggies are a prime example, since they have so much wear and tear during the time they are used. Generally by the time you have bought it and then paid to have it serviced it is not worthwhile.

Car seats are another example. Here the danger is that they may have been involved in an accident and the fixing strap weakened without you realising it. If the model is still current you can buy the seat itself secondhand and buy a new fixing kit. Mattresses are best avoided, especially if the plastic cover is split. They can be very difficult to clean properly. The same goes for wicker cribs and rush Moses baskets.

Most baby clothes can be bought secondhand. The only exception here is shoes. These need to be measured when buying, and leather in particular moulds itself to the wearer's feet.

Of course if you know the person selling the item then that will make buying much easier. If a friend offers you a buggy or car seat you will know how old it is and the sort of wear it is likely to have had. Buying from a stranger is slightly different.

WHERE TO BUY SECONDHAND

Local papers are a very good source of secondhand equipment, but you will have to be prepared to make 'phone calls and go out and look at things. Bear in mind that it can be very difficult to refuse to buy something

when you are standing in someone else's home!
Secondhand shops, boot fairs and local markets often have baby equipment for sale, and you may find an informal 'shop' set up by a local mother who buys and sells in her own home for commission. Local mother and toddler groups, playgroups, and nursery schools often have nearly new tables at their meetings. Some groups run nearly new sales. These are usually run on a commission basis, with everyone bringing along their items and giving a percentage of the selling price to the charity concerned. My local branch of the National Childbirth Trust has two nearly new sales each year, and turns over just over £1,000 each time, which makes profit for the branch and for the people selling. It is also an ideal time for new parents to get together and compare secondhand equipment and clothes.

HIRING EQUIPMENT

Items that are only used occasionally, such as travel cots or carriers, can sometimes be hired. This cuts costs considerably and allows you to try out equipment before buying too. If space is tight it also means you don't have to store items you only want to use once or twice a year. You may be able to hire equipment from friends, or from local groups such as the NCT, or mother and toddler groups. Some independent nursery stores will also hire equipment.

6 STORING AND CLEANING BABY EQUIPMENT

Once an item of baby equipment is no longer needed it is very tempting to put it into the loft and forget about it. However, this often means that two or three years later when you get it down for baby number two to use it is at best very dirty or at worst completely unusable.

It is worth the effort to clean, repair and pack baby things away properly, so that they are ready for use when needed. How each item is cleaned depends mainly on what it is made of.

STORING AND CLEANING

MATERIAL	TREATMENT
Plastic E.g. baths, seats, potties, buckets, cup, plates etc.	Wash well in warm soapy water. Then make up a sterilising tablet in the strength used for sterilising bottles. Wet a cloth in this, wring out and wipe over the plastic item. Slight scratches can be improved by rubbing with a damp cloth dipped in bicarbonate of soda. If this fails, try using a little brass cleaner. Work it into the scratch then rinse it off. Dry and store in a cardboard box in a loft, garage or cellar.
Fabrics E.g. blankets, crib covers etc.	Removable linings and covers should be removed and washed. Dry well, iron lightly and once completely dry, fold and pack away in a strong box lined with tissue paper.

MATERIAL	TREATMENT
Metal, painted or chrome E.g. pushchair and pram frames, highchair frames, stands for carrycots, baths, seat frames.	Wash and dry well before storing. Chrome in particular is prone to rust spots. Wipe existing spots with a damp cloth dipped in bicarbonate of soda. Dry and then smear with a thin film of vaseline or oil before storing. Chrome that has been stored without vaseline or oil on it can be cleaned with a specialist chrome cleaner available from car accessory shops, or a silver cleaner. Also cover any metal ends or joints on painted metal work with vaseline before storing. Chips in painted metal should be rubbed down and touched up before storing. Put spare or loose screws and knobs in an envelope, label clearly, and store with the item they belong to.
Fixed fabric finishes E.g. cord pushchair seats and pram bodies, fabric linings for carrycots and cribs, fabric mattresses.	Fixed fabric finishes like pushchair seats need to be cleaned in situ. Some seating is specially finished to prevent stains and spills penetrating. These can be wiped over or scrubbed if necessary with warm soapy water. Soft cord pram bodies can be vacuumed lightly if necessary and cleaned with a cloth dipped in warm water to which pure soap flakes have been added. Wipe clean with a cloth dipped in clean water and allow to dry *completely* before storing. Dry with the hood up and apron on. Place in a large cardboard box or wrap round with old cloths and sheets before placing in the loft or garage. Avoid storing in a cellar if it is even slightly damp.

MATERIAL	TREATMENT
Soft plastic E.g. high chair seats, interior of carrycots etc.	Wash with warm soapy water. Use an old tootbrush to get into corners and seams. Dry well before storing.
Wheels E.g. on prams and pushchairs.	Use a long-bristled brush dipped in warm soapy water to scrub around wheels. Brush in between the wheels of balloon wheels as small pieces of grit can often become trapped in them. Dry well and then coat metal parts with a little vaseline or oil before storing.

QUICK CLEANING TIPS

1. Wipe the metal parts of the pushchair or pram with a dry cloth if you have been out in the rain. This will prevent rust spots appearing.
2. Allow cord pram hoods and covers to dry before putting the pram/pushchair away. Make sure the hood is up and cover on before drying as they will shrink slightly and be much more difficult to get on otherwise.
3. If your child is often slightly sick it is worth making up a mixture of one pint of warm water plus one teaspoon of bicarbonate of soda. This will clean most surfaces and remove the smell at the same time. Put it in a small plastic bottle designed for spraying plants as this will give a fine mist and avoid over-wetting carpets, cushions and seats. Ideal to keep in the car to help cope with car sickness.
4. Use an old plastic tablecloth under the high chair if your dining room has carpets. Then at the end of the meal just shake off the debris and fold the tablecloth up ready for next time.
5. Mild cream cleaners designed for use in the bath and sink will also remove sticky handmarks from paintwork, plastic and woodwork.

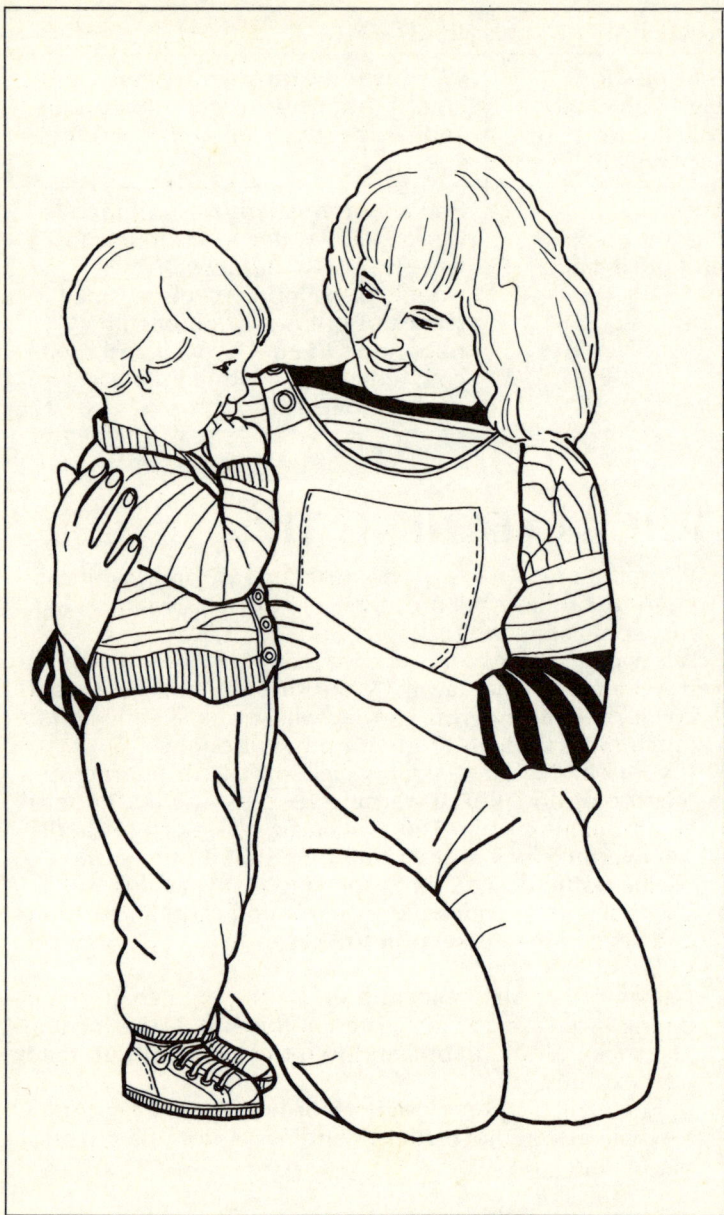

7 SAVING YOUR SANITY

Most parents find there are days when sanity appears to be going out of the window. You swore you would never shout and scream at your toddler, but the day he spreads the jam on himself rather than the bread, or tips the nappy bucket over and then plays with the nappies is the afternoon you give up and want to run away. My worst ever day was when my son and his friend discovered how to strip 'easy strip' wallpaper. By the time I wondered why they were so quiet they had removed the wallpaper from one wall in the bedroom and started on another!

Usually if you can get out of the house for part of each day both you and baby feel better. However, when it rains for days on end and your baby has a cold so you cannot venture out, life can be fraught. Company can lessen the problems and cheer up both you and your baby. Invite another mother round for coffee, lunch or tea. If this is not possible, try some of these rainy day tips.

RAINY DAY TIPS

1. Keep a rainy day box. Put into it toys given for birthdays and Christmas that don't really interest them at the time. Next rainy day allow them to choose a new toy from the box.
2. For slightly older children keep a 'doing' box. Store egg cartons, loo roll inners, paper, sticky shapes etc. in here and use them for making monsters, castles, toys and sticky pictures.
3. Make rainy day cakes. Allow your child to sit in the highchair near you, or if he is old enough to stand on a chair and let him help. Make cakes or biscuits with the emphasis being on letting him join in as much as possible. It may just be that your baby can bang a wooden spoon on the high chair tray but he will still enjoy being with you. As he grows you can let him taste the mixture, play with some biscuit dough, and

eventually help you mix, roll, cut out and put cherries on in pretty patterns.

4. An extra large cardboard box makes a good play house. Help by cutting out windows and doors and playing peep boo through them. Older children will enjoy picnicking in their den.

5. Go swimming at the local pool. Babies can begin after their first innoculations and it won't matter about the rain once you are there.

6. Have a shopping centre picnic. If you cannot stand the house any longer, take a picnic lunch to your nearest shopping centre that is covered in and warm. It's ideal when babies are newly mobile and want space to run around. Go when it's not too busy and there will be room for him to run around and shout as much as he likes.

7. Go for a bus or train ride. It may be completely new to your toddler and can be quite cheap if you just go one stop and back again.

8. Make a scrap book. Cut out your child's favourite pictures from magazines and stick them in a big scrap book so that he can look at them time and again. Let him help in the making.

9. Make music — if you can stand the noise. Let him have a saucepan for a drum and a wooden spoon for a stick. Add a few rice grains safely sealed inside a custard tin or plastic box. Put on a record and dance and play to it.

10. Visit the local library. Many have story telling sessions for mothers and toddlers and often they have lovely bright baby books to look at too.

11. Find out where your local mother and toddler club is and go along to visit. Even a small baby enjoys the company of other babies.

12. With older children, play special rainy day games. Try a colour trail. Walk round the house searching for everything of one colour. Or make a 'feely' box. Seal a cardboard box at one end and cut a flap in the side. You hide something in the box and your child has to feel through the flap to guess what it is. Even quite a small child will enjoy feeling for his teddy or a banana. Older children will enjoy the textures and shapes of things, and you can use the game to help them develop their vocabulary.

13. With toddlers go puddle jumping. Wrap up well and

put the lunch in the oven. Then go out and enjoy the rain. Come back to a hot meal and a warm house.

14. For older children, keep a button jar full of large old buttons. You can thread large ones onto wool with a bodkin, sort them into colours in yoghurt pots, hide them and search for them.

TRAVELLING TIPS

Tiny babies usually travel quite well since they are prepared to sleep almost anywhere. Toddlers and above may well become quite bored, but if you are well prepared and have plenty of games to play it needn't be too bad. The worst age is the newly crawling baby who wants to be moving and exploring. It's essential to break journeys down into short hops, and allow time for energetic games while out of the car. Travelling by train or plane at least allows them to move around while in motion, but in a car they do need to be strapped in.

Dress your child in loose comfortable clothes when travelling. If they need to look very smart upon arrival take their best clothes and change them just before you arrive. Opt for a T-shirt plus soft top so that you can undress them if it is hot. Avoid tight clothes, belts and stiff collars. Take plenty of spare clothes too in case drinks and food are spilt.

Often small titbits of food and non-sugary drinks will bribe your child into sitting in the car just a little longer and alleviate the boredom. Choose fruits, biscuits, little packets of raisins, sticks of cheese, and miniature sandwiches. Avoid chocolate which melts and becomes sticky very quickly, and sugary fizzy drinks which don't really quench their thirst.

A play tray fitted to the car seat will allow little ones to play with a few toys without constantly dropping them. Put a box of favourite toys in the back, but check to make sure there are none that can be swallowed and no sharp pieces or pointed ends.

Music sometimes helps, and a tape of nursery rhymes or action songs can cheer up a fretful baby.

On a two day/one night coach trip to the Pyrenees with two-year-old Sam we took a surprise bag. Inside were a whole range of little presents each wrapped individually. They ranged from little cartons of juice, packets of raisins, little cheesey biscuits, crisps, an apple etc. to miniature toys such as a magic writing slate, a book, a pretend plastic camera etc. Every time boredom struck we got out the goody bag and allowed Sam to choose the next present. He enjoyed unwrapping them and hit of the trip was a miniature hairdryer set. He spent the next couple of hours offering to do the hair of most of the other passengers on the coach!

ENTERTAINING AN ILL CHILD

Most very small babies generally sleep through an illness. When they are awake often all they want is to be cuddled and fed. However, once they get a little older they are often fretful and need constant attention while ill. Often it is the really minor illnesses that make the greatest demands on the parents: when they are ill enough to need extra attention but not ill enough to sleep all the time.

It is worth remembering that while ill, children generally regress a little. You may well find that he needs to be spoon fed, even though he can manage to feed himself. Or he may want to play with more babyish toys, or simpler games while he is off colour.

Entertaining an ill child can be demanding. Often making a special bed on the sofa allows him to watch what is going on and feel part of the family, while still ensuring that he can comfortably drop off to sleep when he needs to. A travel cot will be ideal for under ones who need to be restrained from falling off the sofa. It is almost impossible to keep a small child in bed, so just use his bed or cot as a base and let him play near it. Encourage him when tired to climb in for a little sleep. Keep games simple and help him to play. Favourite tapes or records and television programmes will help pass the time, but he may well need you to sit and watch with him. Familiar favourite books and stories will help too.

It's often worth changing the place you use as his base during the day. He will get very bored with his surroundings, so arrange to spend some time upstairs or in another room. As long as he is not infectious he may enjoy a walk in his pushchair or a ride in the car just for the change of scenery.

If you put away baby toys like rattles or activity centres, it is worth getting them out now as often ill children will enjoy playing with this sort of toy. Sometimes it helps to pretend that his favourite teddy or doll is ill too. This allows you to talk about how he feels and to pop teddy or doll into his own cot to be looked after.

Variety helps, and he may well become very bored with you all the time. So a friend to visit (once he is no longer infectious) or a special visit from a grandparent will help you both survive.

TWENTY-FIVE WAYS TO AMUSE YOUR CHILD

1. Sit a baby in his bouncing chair where he can watch you work, and talk to him as you go. NB Never leave him on a worktop or table as he may bounce off.
2. Fix a mobile above the changing mat to help distract him while you are changing his nappy.
3. Sit him opposite a mirror. A full length mirror is ideal as he can safely sit on the floor in his bouncing chair while you take time to get dressed or make the beds.
4. Take a walk to feed the ducks. Even small babies enjoy regular walks and they learn a lot about the world as you go.
5. Invite other mothers round. Tiny babies enjoy company even if they are really too small to play with each other.
6. Make a sock monster. Put a clean sock on your hand with the heel uppermost. Stick paper cut-outs on for eyes and make your thumb and fingers work the mouth.

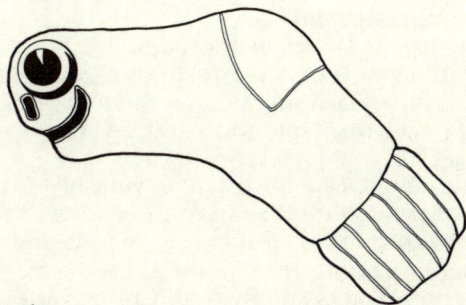

Sock monster

7. Have a bath together. Even if it is the middle of the afternoon a warm bath with plenty of bubbles, toys and watery games can break the spell of a long afternoon trying to amuse a toddler.

8. Keep one kitchen cupboard unlocked and fill it with safe things such as yoghurt pots, wooden spoons, plastic colanders etc. for him to explore and empty out.

9. In warm weather let him sit in the garden and watch the flowers while you do the weeding, put the washing out etc.

10. Once toddling around, let him have a bucket of water and a little watering can to help you water the flowers. NB Always supervise children and water, even when they only have a small amount of it.

11. A paddling pool is ideal for warm weather and the inflatable ones are very cheap to buy.

12. A sandpit is great fun for children from about eighteen months onwards. You only need a small amount of sand, but make sure it is washed sand and not builders' sand which stains clothes and skin. Have strict rules about not throwing sand around, as it can go in their eyes.

13. Make body paints. Mix baby lotion with non-toxic powder paints until it is creamy and brightly coloured. Allow small children to paint their bodies in brightly coloured patterns. Cover the floor with an old plastic tablecloth, and finish with a bath!

14. Make coloured water. Fill old plastic lemonade bottles with water, colour with food colouring, and let them mix the contents and see what happens to the colours. This is definitely a garden game, and you are sure to need dry clothes afterwards, but it can be great fun for two-year-olds upwards.

15. Pouring and measuring will occupy this same age group for a long time. Supply plastic bottles and yoghurt pots, plus a plastic measuring jug. Let them experiment with pouring water from one to the other. Again, messy but fun!

16. Try fingerpaints. Mix poster paint with non-toxic wallpaper paste until it is thick. Then allow them to paint patterns with their hands dipped in the paste.

17. Make paper bag masks. Use the brown paper bags that some supermarkets supply free. Cut eye and mouth holes and decorate to make animals, like elephants or

mice, and monsters. Slip over the head once finished. For three-year-olds upwards, since many small children are very frightened by masks. Also make sure the child knows the difference between paper and plastic bags.

18. Allocate an unused part of the garden as a digging hole. Allow your child to dig there, and let him have a small trowel or fork and a few plastic plant pots.

19. Make a music corner (preferably in the garden for the sake of your ears!) Hang up a few things that make a good noise when struck, e.g. a piece of tubing, a couple of coat hangers, and add some things to bang such as an old biscuit tin. Make shakers using washing up liquid bottles with rice or beans inside. Bigger children can be allowed milk bottles with water in to strike gently to make notes.

20. Keep a dressing up box. Save old scarves, shoes, hats and gaudy clothes, and scout round local jumble sales for suitable dressing up clothes. Several children together enjoy a dressing up box just as much as a child playing alone.

21. Paint a piece of wood or a section of a wall with blackboard paint and supply coloured chalks. Toddlers will enjoy colourful scribbling and older children will draw and write on it.

22. Save old rolls of wallpaper and hang on a piece of string. Unroll as needed and the white side will be uppermost for drawing on. Supply chunky wax crayons for small children and let them sit on the floor and draw on the paper.

23. Sometimes chores appeal to small children. Let them help. Washing the car is often a most popular job with two-year-olds upwards. Give them a cloth and a little bucket of water and plan to change their clothes afterwards.

24. In a similar way, being allowed to wash their toys is often great fun. Help select which toys can be washed, then give them a bucket of warm soapy water and a large old towel. A game best played in the garden!

25. Make a Me picture. Use a piece of wallpaper or a large sheet of brown paper. Lay your child down and draw around him using brightly coloured felt pen. Then let him draw in his own eyes, nose, mouth, clothes etc. Three- and four-year-olds will enjoy measuring how big his hands and feet are, how tall he is etc., and writing

that onto the picture too. Once finished, hang it up in
his bedroom.

TAKING TIME OFF

Parenting is one of the few jobs that offers no holiday or
sick leave, and expects you work twenty-four hours a day
every day of the year. You never stop being a parent, but
all parents need some time away from their children.

It is often hard to leave a tiny baby for the first time.
Usually grandparents and friends are only too willing to
look after him, but it needs a little push before a new
mother can bring herself to leave her baby.

Often it helps if the first time you go out is to
somewhere nearby, so you can come back if needed. Go to
the pub around the corner, or to nearby friends, and make
the time spent away from your baby quite short — just an
hour or so.

Later you may well want to leave the baby all evening. If
you are breast feeding, having a supply of expressed milk
helps. It is worth introducing a bottle quite early on as
some babies will refuse it if given later. Allow breast
feeding to become well established and then occasionally
offer boiled water from a bottle so that your baby knows
how to suck from it. A specially shaped teat helps too. (See
page 54 for more information.) When you do give him
breast milk in a bottle, try to ensure that someone else
offers him the bottle. Often breast-fed babies will not
accept a bottle when they know the breast is available.
Once you know that your baby will not starve without you,
getting out and about makes life easier.

Apart from special occasions it's worth trying to ensure
that you have some free time regularly. It's all too easy to
become submerged by the baby. You may be able to leave
your baby with a grandparent one afternoon each week. Or
try a baby swop; have a friend's baby one morning and she
can have your's another morning. A local childminder may
be available to mind your baby regularly or just
occasionally. Your health visitor should be able to put you
in touch with nearby childminders. Often adult education
centres run crèches, and so too do some health clubs and
fitness centres.

How you find free time will vary. One woman I know

spends Wednesday evening having a sauna. The time afterwards allows her to unwind and do her hair and make up properly without being interrupted or climbed upon by her baby. Another woman has Saturday mornings off. Her husband works long hours during the week and rarely gets to see his children, so he enjoys being in charge one morning a week and she has several hours to do whatever she wants.

It can help to think of the time your baby spends sleeping during the day as extra time for you. It's all too easy to rush around doing all the housework during that hour or two. Then when the baby wakes you are even more tired than when he went to sleep. Instead use that time to do the things you want to do. It may be reading the paper, writing letters, planting seeds or any number of other things. Remember — mothers matter!

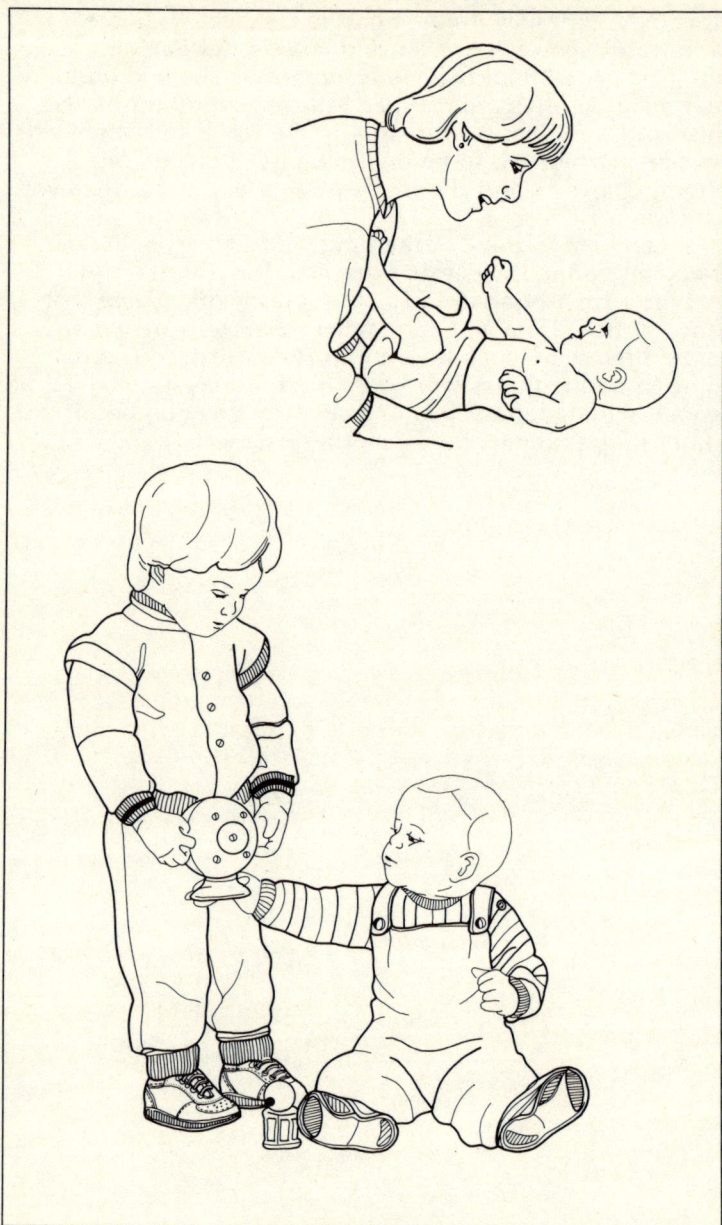

8 BABY HEALTH

IMMUNIZATION

Immunization protects your baby against several diseases that in the past caused at best much misery, and at worst many babies and children to die.

The routine procedure is for a baby to be immunized against certain diseases by a course of injections and drops given by mouth while he is a baby. This is then 'topped up' or boosted by an extra injection just before he starts school. It's often referred to as a pre-school booster. Times for the injections to be given are not rigid, and if your baby is unwell, they can be delayed a week or two. Your doctor and health visitor will give you more details and advise you, but as a rough guide the following table shows the usual timings. It's worth keeping a record of when your baby has his innoculations for future reference.

Many families are concerned about the safety of certain innoculations, particularly whooping cough. Do discuss the pros and cons with your doctor and health visitor. The advice given about having the whooping cough vaccine varies from time to time and it does depend on family history, the baby's birth, and on the health of your baby. Don't underestimate the dangers of whooping cough itself either. If you are advised not to have the whooping cough innoculations, don't forget to have the others.

It's wise to avoid giving innoculations if your baby is unwell. A delay of a few days won't matter. Sometimes the site of the injection is a little sore, and some babies run a slight temperature. Some doctors advise giving a single dose of 'Calpol', or a similar product, just after the innoculation. Ask your GP for her/his advice on this. If your baby does react badly to his innoculation, and runs a very high temperature, cries loudly for a long time or has a convulsion, contact your doctor straight away.

BABY IMMUNIZATION PROGRAMME

TIME	IMMUNIZATION	NAME AND DATE
3–4 months	Injection of diphtheria, whooping cough and tetanus; or diphtheria and tetanus only.	Baby's name: Date given:
	Drops given by month for polio.	Baby's name: Date given:
5–6 months	Triple injection: diphtheria whooping cough and tetanus; or diphtheria and tetanus only.	Baby's name: Date given:
	Polio drops.	Baby's name: Date given:
9–11 months	Triple injection: diphtheria whooping cough and tetanus; or diphtheria and tetanus only.	Baby's name: Date given:
	Polio drops.	Baby's name: Date given:
15–18 months	Immunization against measles by injection.	Baby's name: Date given:
5 years	Pre-school booster of diphtheria, whooping cough and tetanus.	Child's name: Date given:
	Polio drops.	Child's name: Date given:
At secondary school age	German measles by injection for girls only.	Child's name: Date given:
	BCG testing.	Child's name: Date given:

CHILDHOOD ILLNESSES

The very expression 'childhood illnesses' sounds quite unimportant and harmless. Indeed, they generally are. Most children bounce back from sickness quite quickly. It's true that they seem to suffer far less than adults unfortunate enough to suffer one of these childhood illnesses. However, when your child is ill, it can be very worrying. It's hard work too, with broken nights and demanding days. Thankfully there's a limited number of common illnesses to cope with, and they don't usually re-occur. (At least not in the same child!)

It's worth keeping a note of who had what when. Looking back, it can be hard to remember, especially once you have more than one child. Knowing that your child has had certain diseases at least eliminates them from future diagnosis.

Also look at the section on 'Entertaining an Ill Child' on pages 132–3.

MAIN CHILDHOOD ILLNESSES

CHICKEN POX	CHILD'S NAME:	DATE:
SIGNS AND SYMPTOMS	INFECTIOUS PERIOD	NURSING
Your child may be a bit below par or extra tired. Often, though, there is no warning. Blistery spots appear, usually on the trunk first, and spread rapidly. They are very itchy and if they become infected, small	Incubation takes two to three weeks. The disease is at its most infectious just before the spots appear. Many schools will not allow a child to return until all the little scabs left after the blisters have gone. Others	Often this is surprisingly mild. Your child may be irritated by the itching more than anything else. Calamine lotion dabbed on the spots often helps. Rest, plenty of fluids and extra attention are

SIGNS AND SYMPTOMS	INFECTIOUS PERIOD	NURSING
scars can be left afterwards.	allow return once no new spots appear.	usually all that is needed. Use paracetamol and sponging to control temperature and ease discomfort.
GERMAN MEASLES	CHILD'S NAME:	DATE:
Pink mottly rash. Usually it begins behind the ears and spreads to the trunk. Sometimes comes and goes very quickly. You may be able to feel the small glands at the back of the neck just below the hairline. These are often swollen and tender.	This takes two to three weeks to appear and is infectious for about five days.	A mild illness but worth having diagnosed simply because of the dangers to pregnant mothers. Avoid taking your child out, even shopping, since the dangers to a newly pregnant woman are so great. If your baby has been in contact with anyone pregnant, it's worth letting them know as they can see their GP to check their immunity.
MEASLES	CHILD'S NAME:	DATE:
This usually starts with a cold and runny nose, and a	It takes one to two weeks for the disease to develop	Measles makes children very poorly. Your baby

SIGNS AND SYMPTOMS	INFECTIOUS PERIOD	NURSING
rising temperature. The rash begins behind the ears and spreads rapidly. The spots are dark pinky red.	and your child may be ill for three to four days before the spots come out. He will remain infectious for between ten and fourteen days.	may develop a cough as well as running a very high temperature. It can lead to other infectious such as bronchitus or middle ear infection. He will need lots of attention and plenty of fluids. Call your GP who will be able to check for secondary infections and prescribe antibiotics if necessary. Rarely, measles may cause convulsions, and there is a very slight possibility of inflammation of the brain, so don't underestimate the disease. Use paracetamol and sponging to control temperature and ease discomfort.

MUMPS	CHILD'S NAME:	DATE:
SIGNS AND SYMPTOMS	INFECTIOUS PERIOD	NURSING
Your child may simply seem a little run down and extra grumpy at first. Swelling of the face is the definite sign. The area from just underneath the ear to round under the jaw bone is usually swollen and very tender. Often children find opening their mouth quite difficult and swallowing may be painful.	This takes between two and four weeks to develop. It's at its most infectious before the swelling begins.	This is a jolly uncomfortable disease and older children are often quite distressed by the swelling. Eating is very difficult. Milky drinks are easier, but avoid fruit juices which often sting when swallowed. Use a children's painkiller as necessary, and keep him warm and comfortable. Some children suffer deafness after mumps, so if you think he may not be hearing, return to your GP to double check.

COPING WITH A FEVER

Babies and young children can run high temperatures very rapidly. It is worth using a paracetamol product designed for babies to reduce the temperature and ease pain and discomfort.

Combine this with sponging a baby's skin to help bring the temperature down. Undress your baby down to his nappy, and sponge him down with lukewarm (**not** cold) water. Let the water evaporate from his body rather than drying him with a towel. Once you have brought his temperature down he is likely to be more comfortable and may be able to sleep.

Don't ignore a high temperature in a baby. It can lead to febrile convulsions or indicate an illness coming on. However, babies' temperatures can increase and drop rapidly and often paracetamol and sponging will help a great deal. If worried, always double-check with your GP.

Do not give aspirin-based products to children under 12 years unless on a doctor's advice.

BASIC FIRST AID

Children are naturally inquisitive and adventurous, so accidents do happen. But try to make your home and garden as safe as possible to minimise the dangers. As well as checking the house, remember the garage or garden shed with its lawn mower, shears and weedkiller, and the front gate onto the road.

As early as possible, teach your children why things are dangerous, and make rules that they never touch knives or scissors, for example, or never open bottles without asking first. Even so, assume that when they are pre-occupied with friends and imaginative games that they will forget everything in their enthusiasm to find out about the world around them.

Equip a basic first aid kit, and keep it handy where everyone knows where it is, and prepare yourself by learning about basic first aid.

Nothing can replace a proper practical first aid course. Once you become a parent, you are more likely to have to deal with minor accidents and prompt action can minimise problems. Even if you don't have time for a full course, many first aid organisations now run one-off sessions where a particular aspect of first aid is covered.

If several parents get together, it's often possible to organise an evening specially for 'family first aid'. Look in your local telephone directory under Red Cross or St John's Ambulance.

In the event of an accident, however minor, it's vital to keep calm. Use the relaxation techniques you learned at antenatal classes to help. If you are calm, your baby will be less upset. One mother did this so efficiently when her son cut the top off his finger, that in the ambulance on the way to hospital, the little boy was calmly pointing out the cows and sheep as they sped along the country lanes! The mother meanwhile, was striving to keep up the general flow of conversation while holding onto the top of the finger, and worrying about having it sewn back on.

First aid is meant to be just that; initial aid to deal with the problem until you can see your doctor or get to hospital. So do just what's needed immediately and then seek help. It may seem quicker to drive your child to hospital than call an ambulance, but it's impossible to drive and comfort a distressed child. Ambulance men and women will be able to give prompt comprehensive first aid, and care for your child en route to the hospital too.

BLEEDING

Many children are very alarmed by even small amounts of blood and need very calm, matter-of-fact treatment. Most cuts will simply need cleaning, and a plaster or bandage. Major bleeding is more serious. Check first for foreign bodies in the wound. Apply direct pressure on the wound, cover with a clean cloth, bandage or even a wad of kitchen towel, and put on steady even pressure.

For a wound with foreign bodies in, such as glass or grit, apply pressure around the wound not on it. Then consult your doctor or take the child to hospital, or call an ambulance.

If possible, raise that part of the body too. The bleeding should slow down and you can then apply a firm bandage with a good pad of lint over the site of the wound.

If the bleeding continues, or starts up again once you remove the pressure take the child to the doctor or hospital, or call an ambulance.

Bleeding from the mouth is often quite copious. A bitten lip or tongue can bleed a great deal. A wad of cotton wool placed in the mouth and pressed against the wound will usually help.

BURNS AND SCALDS

If a child's clothes are on fire, lay the child on the ground immediately with the flames uppermost. Smother the flames with water, a towel, blanket or coat — whatever is to hand. If nothing is available, lie flat on the child to smother the flames. Avoid using synthetic fabrics as these can melt in the heat.

Immerse the affected part in cold water immediately. This may well mean sitting your child in the bath or sink, or simply holding a burnt finger in a bowl of water. Keep it there until the pain subsides or for a good ten minutes. If the burn is over a large area, or likely to be very deep, call an ambulance and remain with the affected part in cold water until it arrives.

Don't be tempted to put anything on the burn: it will only have to be removed before the burn can be assessed and treated.

Small burns need the cooling treatment and then simply covering with a clean dry bandage. His body will do the healing without extras like ointments. Double check with your doctor that no further treatment is needed.

CHOKING

This can be very frightening and it's something that small children seem to do quite often. Thankfully, the body's coughing response usually clears the obstruction. If it doesn't, you will have to help. Hold the baby with his back to you across your lap with his head tilted down. With a small baby you can hold them upside down. Give a couple of hard sharp slaps to his back between the shoulder blades to try and dislodge the object. If this fails and your child cannot breathe, reach into the back of his mouth and try to locate the object using your finger. With a toddler or older child, you can also try to force the object out by sitting him on your lap, facing away from you; put your arms around him just above waist level and grasp your hands together. Give a sudden sharp squeeze, in and up just between the ribs, and below the breastbone. This forces air up the tubes and may clear the obstruction.

If the obstruction will not clear, or if you are unsure if the object has come out completely, call an ambulance.

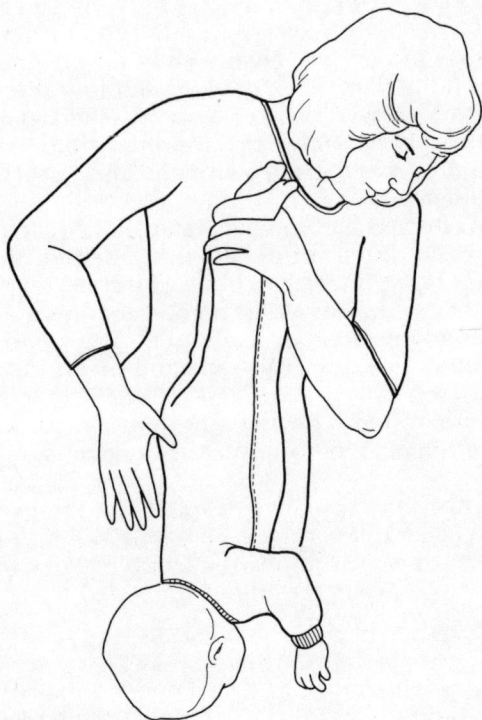

Hold a small baby upside-down to help clear an obstruction.

EARS AND NOSES

Only try to remove a foreign body if you can grasp it firmly and not risk damaging the child's ear or nose, or pushing it in further. Take the child to the doctor or hospital where they have special instruments available.

EYES

Sand, grass or bits of grit in the eye feel very uncomfortable, and can do damage if left. Often you can remove it using a corner of a clean piece of cotton, but you really need your child's co-operation in keeping still for this. You can wrap a baby in a large bath towel to pin his arms down and stop him wriggling. Then sit on a sofa with him tucked under your arm so that his head is on your lap and his legs on the sofa. This is a useful technique for putting eye drops and cream in too.

An older child can be helped to use a water bath. Fill an egg cup with cold water and put your child's eye onto it. He will need to bend down as if he were looking in it. Then lift the egg cup up as he stands up, so the water flows into the eye. Persuade him to open his eye and blink a little. Wrap a towel around his shoulders as some is sure to spill.

If you cannot remove the object or the eye is even slightly scratched, see your doctor or go to the hospital.

FALLS

Most children bounce back from falls and knocks. However, their bones are very soft and they do sometimes damage themselves, so always check them over after a fall. A cuddle and a few words of comfort while you feel the affected part will also help them recover more quickly. If the affected part is swollen and tender, and he cannot move it or put any weight on it, there may be a 'greenstick' fracture. These are common in children, and very difficult to diagnose. Check with your doctor, or take him to hospital. Often, only an X-ray can distinguish between a sprain and a fracture of this kind.

More major fractures tend to be obvious, with the affected part obviously mishapen or lying at a strange angle. Your child will be unable to use or move it without great pain. Call an ambulance and don't move the child if you can avoid it. Even if the accident has happened on the beach or park, it is better to keep him still and send someone else to ring for an ambulance. Ambulances carry inflatable splints, and gas and oxygen, which make moving him much safer and less painful.

If your child bangs his head during a fall, keep an eye on

him. If he is dizzy, drowsy, vomits or cannot see clearly, take him to your doctor or hospital. Keep him awake and keep talking to him. Often an overnight hospital stay is recommended simply for observation, even if there is no fracture.

If the fall is so serious that the child is knocked unconscious, check that the child is breathing and has a pulse. The best place to feel the pulse is under the jaw below the ear lobe. Then place your child in the recovery position and call an ambulance immediately.

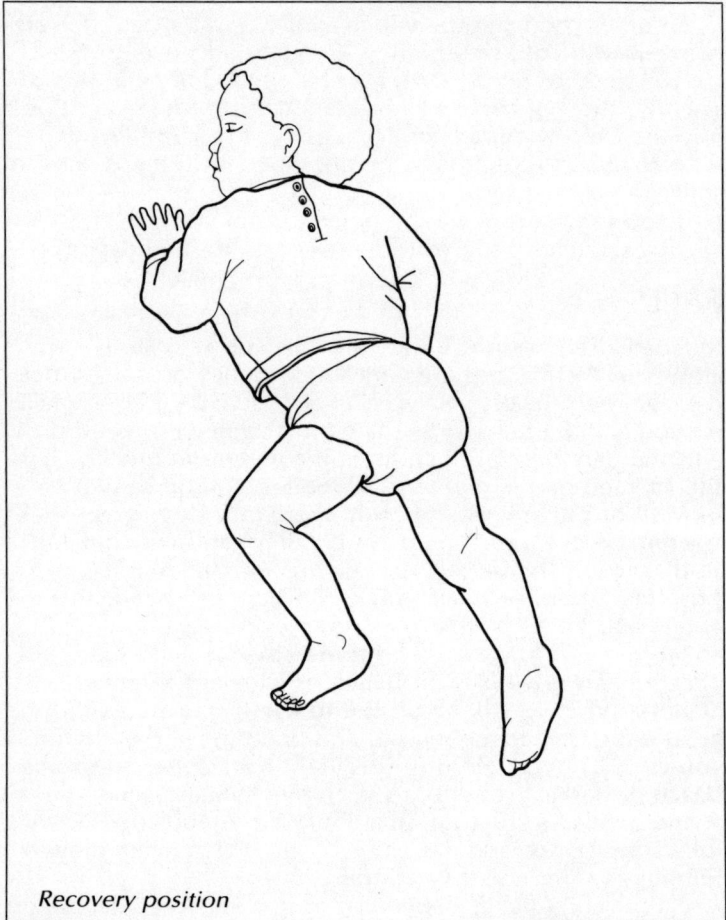

Recovery position

MOUTH-TO-MOUTH RESUSCITATION

If a child is not breathing, you must start mouth-to-mouth resuscitation immediately.

1. Check that there is nothing in the mouth to block the airway.
2. Tuck the child's head back to open the airway.

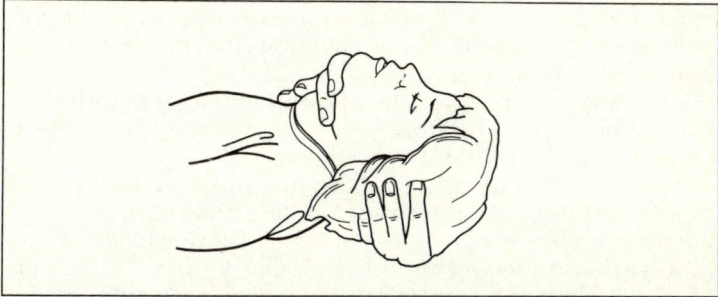

3. With your mouth over his nose and mouth, breathe in gently, take your mouth away and allow the air to be expelled. Do this four times. If breathing has not restarted, continue until he starts breathing on his own, then place him in the recovery position.

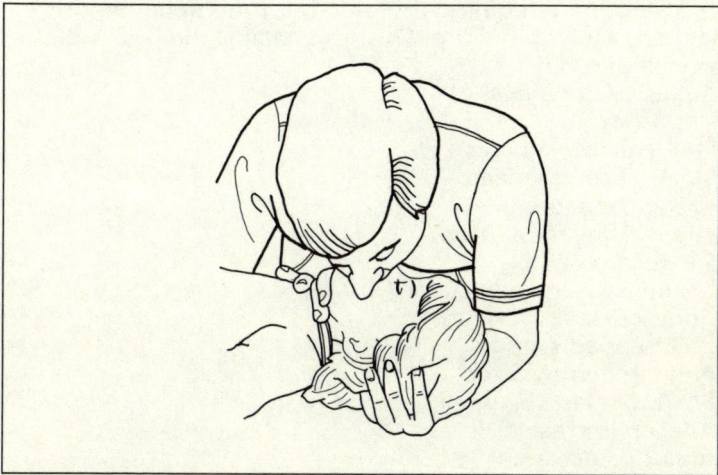

4. Call for an ambulance as early as possible but do not leave the child.

POISONS

Always make sure that medicines and tablets are safely locked away, and check also that household cleaners and other products are well out of reach. An amazing number of everyday household cleaners and products are highly poisonous too. Even alcohol and tobacco can kill a small child. Take great care to keep all possible poisons out of reach and safely locked up. If your child does eat or drink pills, berries, toilet blocks or anything similar which is non-caustic, remove any remaining parts of it from his mouth, and try to make him sick. Put two fingers into the back of his throat and hold him head down so that if he is sick, he will not inhale it.

The exception here is anything that will have burned his mouth and throat as it went down, like bleach, most household cleaners and paint solvent. These will simply burn again on the way up. Instead, give your child a drink of milk and wash his mouth out with water or milk.

In either case, take your child (and the substance, or the bottle if there is none left) to hospital immediately, or ring for an ambulance.

FIRST AID KIT

It is sensible to equip a first aid kit for the home before you are likely to need it. This list contains the basics that you should buy.
Adhesive dressings.
Cotton wool.
Sterile gauze squares.
Small gauze bandage.
Crêpe bandage.
Tubular finger bandage.
Safety pins.
Triangular bandage.
Adhesive tape (surgical).
Blunt-ended scissors.
Blunt-ended tweezers.
Soap for cleaning wounds.
Antiseptic cream.
Junior paracetamol.

SOURCES OF HELP

There is a wide range of voluntary and official agencies around to help with parenting and family life. Your GP's notice board, local papers or telephone directory may list local branches of these, but if not, contact the main offices listed here, who will be able to put you in touch with your nearest branch.

ASSOCIATION FOR IMPROVEMENTS IN MATERNITY
SERVICES (AIMS)
67 Leanard Road, London, SE20

ASSOCIATION FOR POSTNATAL ILLNESS
7 Gowan Avenue, Fulham, London, SW6   01 731 4867

BRITISH RED CROSS SOCIETY
9, Grosvenor Crescent, London, SW1X 7EJ   01 235 5454

COELIAC SOCIETY
PO Box 181, London, NW2 2QY

COMPASSIONATE FRIENDS
6 Denmark Street, Bristol, BS1 5DQ   0272 292778

CRYSIS
Zita Thornton, National Co-ordinator, 63 Putney Road,
Freezywater, Enfield, Middlesex.   Lea Valley   716645

FOUNDATION OF THE STUDY OF INFANT DEATHS
5th Floor, 4 Grosvenor Place, London, SW1X 7HD
01 235 1721

GINGERBREAD
35 Wellington Street, London, WC2E 7BN   01 240 0953

HEALTH EDUCATION COUNCIL
78 New Oxford Street, London, WC1A 1AH   01 637 1881

LA LÈCHE LEAGUE OF GREAT BRITAIN
PO Box BM 3434, London, WC1 3XX   01 242 1278

MEET-A-MUM-ASSOCIATION
3 Woodside Avenue, South Norwood, London, SE25
5DW   01 654 3137

MENCAP
National Centre, 123 Golden Lane, London, EC1Y 0RT
01 253 9433

NATIONAL ASSOCIATION FOR MATERNAL AND CHILD WELFARE
1 South Audley Street, London, W1Y 6JS

NATIONAL CHILDBIRTH TRUST
9 Queensborough Terrace, Bayswater, London, W2
3TB   01 221 3833

NATIONAL CHILDMINDING ASSOCIATION
204/206 High Street, Bromley, Kent, BR1 1PP   01 464 6164

NATIONAL COUNCIL FOR ONE-PARENT FAMILIES
255 Kentish Town Road, London, NW5 2LK   01 267 1361

NATIONAL ECZEMA SOCIETY
Tavistock House, Tavistock Square, London, WC1H
9SR   01 387 9681

NATIONAL SOCIETY FOR THE PREVENTION OF CRUELTY TO CHILDREN
67 Saffron Hill, London, EC1N 8RF   01 242 1626

ORGANISATION FOR PARENTS UNDER STRESS (OPUS)
106 Godstone Road, Whyteleafe, Croydon, Surrey, CR30
0EB   01 654 0469

PARENTS ANONYMOUS
6 Manor Gardens, London, N7 6LA   01 263 8918

PRE-SCHOOL PLAYGROUPS ASSOCIATION
Alford House, Aveline Street, London, SE11 5DH
01 582 1924

ST JOHN AMBULANCE
1 Grosvenor Crescent, London, SW1X 7EF   01 235 5231

THE SPASTICS SOCIETY
12 Park Crescent, London, W1N 4EQ   01 636 5020

STILLBIRTH AND NEONATAL DEATH SOCIETY (SANDS)
Argyle House, 29–31 Euston Road, London, NW1 2SD
01 833 2851

TWINS AND MULTIPLE BIRTHS ASSOCIATION
Mrs D. Hoseason, 54 Broad Lane, Hampton, Middlesex,
TW12 3BG

BABY'S RECORD CHART

Name	
Born on	
Time	
At	
Weight	
Baptised/Christened on	
at	
First Smile	
First Laugh	
Rolled over for First Time	
Sat Up	
First Tooth Appeared	
First Foods	
Crawled	
First Steps Taken	
First Words	

ESSENTIAL TELEPHONE NUMBERS

Midwife	
Doctor	
Health Visitor	
Baby Clinic	
Local Hospital	
Dentist	
Childminder	
DHSS	
Friends	

INDEX